Natural Body, Natural Shape

Natural Body, Natural Shape

Develop a Strong Self-Image, Good Health, & Ageless Grace & Beauty Through Yoga

Barbara B. Moroney

SWING-HI PRESS
AURORA, COLORADO

Although the author and publisher have made every effort to ensure the accuracy and completeness of information contained in this book, we assume no responsibility for errors, inaccuracies, omissions, or any inconsistency herein. Any slights of people, places, or organizations are unintentional.

Portia Nelson, *There's a Hole in My Sidewalk,* "AUTOBIOGRAPHY IN FIVE SHORT CHAPTERS," copyright © 1993, reprinted by permission of Beyond Words Publishing, Inc., Hillsboro, Oregon, U.S.A. Quote from *The Concise Light on Yoga,* copyright 1980 by George Allen & Unwin Ltd. Quotes from *Tuesdays with Morrie: An Old Man, a Young Man, and Life's Greatest Lesson,* copyright 1997 by Mitch Albom. Quotes from *Having Our Say: The Delany Sisters' First 100 Years,* copyright 1993 by Amy Hill Hearth, Sarah Louise Delany, and Annie Elizabeth Delany.

Cartoon illustrations by Anna-Maria Crum.
Yoga illustrations by Mark Bremmer.

First printing 2003

ISBN 0-9724335-4-6
LCCN 2002112810

Acknowledgments

The motivation for writing this book came from the profound joy and benefit I have received from practicing yoga and qi gong. The desire to develop a new and healthy relationship with my body evolved naturally from the regular practice of these disciplines.

I am deeply grateful to all of my teachers and my teachers' teachers for the valuable practices I have learned from them. I am especially grateful to Debra Ann Robinson (yoga) and Zhu Xilin (qi gong), two extraordinarily gifted teachers. Special thanks also to my first yoga teacher, Isabelle (Isa) D'Onofrio.

Some authors write six or seven books in nine years. I have written six or seven versions of the same book over that period. Having never written anything before, I had no idea how hard it is to translate your ideas into the written word. One has to understand the rules of grammar for the translation to be precise. I want to thank my wonderful friend Nicole Sperekas for reading and critiquing the content and grammar of my work from the very first draft to the final revision. I am also grateful for her friendly support and counsel during the whole process of bringing my book to completion. My friend Merlin Stone also critiqued my work and gave me valuable insight.

I am grateful to Steve Berger, editor of one of my earlier versions, who helped point the way toward my final goal and just as importantly, patiently coaxed me into taking the big step of showing my manuscript to a stranger.

Several versions later I took my final draft to Tom and Marilyn Ross of About Books, Inc. I appreciate the professional, warm support I received from them and their staff. They expertly guided me through the maze of self-publishing and helped transform my manuscript into the final product—a book I finally have in print.

The illustrations of the yoga and qi gong postures in the book were drawn from models. I am grateful for the time they took from their busy schedules to pose for me. Many thanks to Ashlee Dunn, Debra Ann Robinson, Jeanne Ann Walter, Lura Williams, Steve Koehler, Suzanna Del Vecchio, and Zhu Xilin.

Debra Ann and Zhu helped me with the instructions for guiding my readers into the yoga poses I present in the book. Isabelle Hutton, reflexologist and massage therapist, helped me with my Footprint Exercises. Debra Ann, Zhu, and Isabelle have a profound understanding of their work. Any errors in the presentations are mine.

Finally, I want to express my love and appreciation to my husband Bob for being my love and companion and for his unwavering support and encouragement of my project. My love also goes to my son Neill, who is my heart, and to my father, whose unconditional love is a gift. My sister Margaret, my sister-in-spirit Lynn, my soul sister Delores, and all of my friends who are in the pages of this book as much as I am. Thank you for being who you are.

This book is dedicated in loving memory of my mother.

Table of Contents

Introduction

I gazed into the mirror. My reflection showed a body that was trim and moderately athletic in a new tennis outfit with a short, pleated skirt. I turned to view my profile from the left, then the right. As I turned, my gaze hardened into a glare as it zeroed in and locked onto my stomach. I focused disappointment and frustration into that glare for several moments. Then, breaking the momentary trance-like communication with my stomach, check-over complete, I grabbed my tennis racquet and headed for the door.

It was the summer of 1993. I had sold my business in February and decided I would begin to make up for the lack of playfulness and fun in my life by devoting the summer to playing tennis. During the drive to the tennis courts, the glare I had leveled at my stomach lingered in my mind. It was like an internal spotlight that never turned itself off, even when I wasn't fully conscious of what I was doing to myself. I hated my stomach. The rest of my body was passable. But my stomach stuck out. Even at my lowest summer weight, it was round instead of fashionably flat, with the hard and rubbery consistency of an oversized Spalding handball. The tennis skirt, with its elastic waistband and pleats, emphasized its ugly bulk.

I knew I wasn't fat, but I never felt thin enough and always struggled to eat as little as possible. Struggle, struggle, struggle. My body was an adversary. It ate things I didn't want. It was tired and lazy when I felt I should be jogging. But most importantly, it would not, no matter what I did, turn into the ideal body I wanted. Carefully constructed over the years, my ideal body looked like this:

Julie Christie's nose (*Dr. Zhivago*, 1968), a 21-inch waist (probably Barbie), and a stomach in line with the front tips of my hipbones (magazine ads for lingerie).

1

Over the years my body remained essentially the same: Boris Yeltsin's nose (my Russian heritage), a 21-inch waist in my dreams, and a rubber-ball stomach.

As the passage of time took me farther and farther away from it, I also wanted my twenty-five-year-old body back. My ideal body image was a Dorian Gray reflection in reverse. It stayed young while I grew old.

The burden of this ideal body, growing monstrously with the added unresolved problem of aging, felt like a ball and chain dragging along wherever I went. The image dictated my daily wardrobe (there are thin-stomach clothes and fat-stomach clothes), my diet, my posture, and my daily mental outlook (thin-stomach days start off sunnier than fat-stomach days).

I had been at war with my body for as long as I could remember. This war—waged with diet, exercise, and cosmetic surgery—was the unhappy means I had adopted to transform my body shape into the ideal image of how I wanted it to look. Like a disillusioned soldier, I was weary and no longer sure of the cause for which I was fighting. I wanted to find peace in love and self-acceptance. Whatever all of that meant.

What, I wondered, does it mean to love and totally accept one's self? Should you never try to make yourself look better? Should you not dye your hair when you start to go gray? Should you not try to lose weight if you are overweight? And when are you overweight? Should you never have cosmetic surgery? What is the happy medium between excessive self-criticism and a healthy desire to improve your appearance? How would you know when you found it?

The sale of my business, together with my daily practice of yoga, gave me the time and the focus to consider this dilemma in depth.

So, in the fall of 1993, I began a journey of exploration into my relationship with my body during which I have examined many of the insecurities, fears, and judgments that had created an image I could never live up to. It is a journey that continues to date. Not only am I not at the end of this journey, I am not sure there is an end to it. However, I have discovered a more natural body shape that is different from the ideal image I had struggled with for most of my life. This natural body shape is healthier, stronger, more balanced

2

than the one I had twenty years ago, and reflects the benefits of regular yoga practice. Along the way I have learned some fundamental truths about self-acceptance and how to create a happy relationship with my body that I would like to share with others.

I wrote this book hoping it would inspire other women who, like me, struggle to find self-acceptance and peace with their physical bodies and themselves. In addition to the chronicle of my journey, I have included related exercises for my readers to try. It takes work and dedication to bring about change and while this book can be read without doing any of the exercises, I recommend working with them for a richer experience.

Journal Entry

I sat cross-legged on the floor behind the closed door of my office and began to breathe deeply and evenly to relax. I closed my eyes and visualized the image of how I want to look. Maybe, if I brought it up and looked it straight in the eye, I could release its hold.

I saw a young girl I had once watched perform on the stage of a local theater production. She was very young. She had gorgeous hair and one of the tiniest waists I have ever seen. She looked like a miniature porcelain doll, like my brunette Barbie dolls.

Where did the memory of her come from? Until now, I hadn't consciously thought of this young girl beyond that one time I saw her.

To look like this Barbie doll clone I would have to do something really drastic—maybe saw off a few of my ribs and a piece of my pelvis. I opened my eyes. I pictured a cartoon-like solution of lining my body up on a three-sectioned frame that matches up different heads, torsos, and legs. My cartoon self would feel no pain as I cut out and replaced the middle section with the correct-sized hips, waist, and stomach.

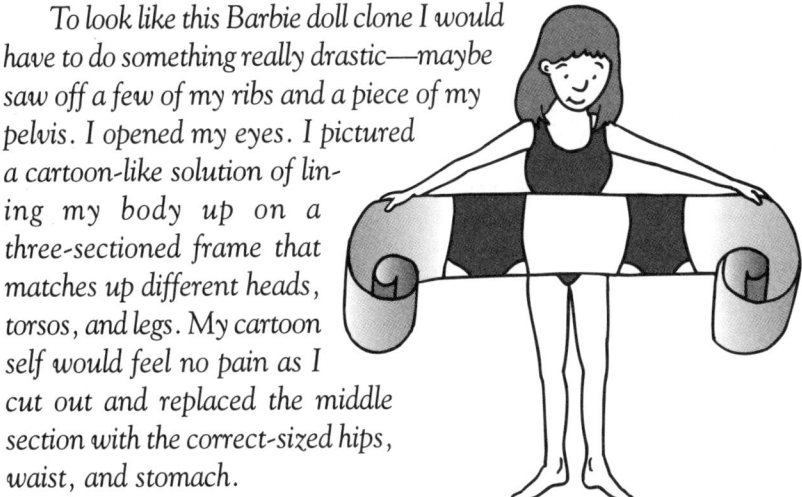

What if I just let go of the image? "I let you go," I said. I felt afraid. A stream of anxious thoughts followed—I can't do that. I'll lose control. I'll gain a hundred pounds and really be fat. Letting the image go felt like setting myself adrift, rudderless in the sea. My body seemed to dissolve into an amorphous mass.

I saw myself attached to the image by a rope that extended from my feet. The rope felt like security. The ideal image was a guidepost, something reassuringly tangible to work toward to be acceptable.

"I love and accept myself as I am," I said. The words had no life force to them. They were like a coil of wire with a broken electrical connection. Like Dickens' Jacob Marley, they were as dead as a doornail.

Ideal Body Image Exercise

1. Sit comfortably in a chair with your feet resting on the floor and parallel to each other. Rest your hands lightly on your thighs.

2. Close your eyes and take a deep breath to relax.

3. Focus your attention on the tips of your nostrils where the breath enters and leaves your body. Breathe deeply and slowly for one minute.

4. Visualize the body you would like to have. Take your time with the visualization, make it as detailed as possible.

5. Mentally compare this ideal image to the body you have. What parts of it match the body you have? What parts do not?

6. How are you attached to this image? To find out, ask yourself, "How am I attached to this image?" Do any visual or auditory clues materialize?

7. Imagine yourself letting the image go. Say aloud, "I let this image go." What do you think and feel when you say this?

8. Open your eyes.

If you had trouble forming a visual picture of your image, go through magazines, watch TV, take note of other women you see. Cut out pictures that represent how you want to look. Draw an outline of your body on paper, using the mirror as a guide.

Visualization Notes

Consider the following questions:

1. How were the physical characteristics of your ideal image different from your real body?

2. How were the physical characteristics of your ideal image the same as your real body?

3. Which characteristics of your ideal body do you think are a realistic goal, given your body type? Which characteristics are not? (You may not know for sure on some of these; answer to the best of your ability for now.)

4. Were you able to visualize your attachment to your image? What did the attachment mean to you? Also describe what you felt when you imagined letting go of the image.

    Record any other significant thoughts and observations, using the page below to describe your experience.

Part 1

Out of Egypt

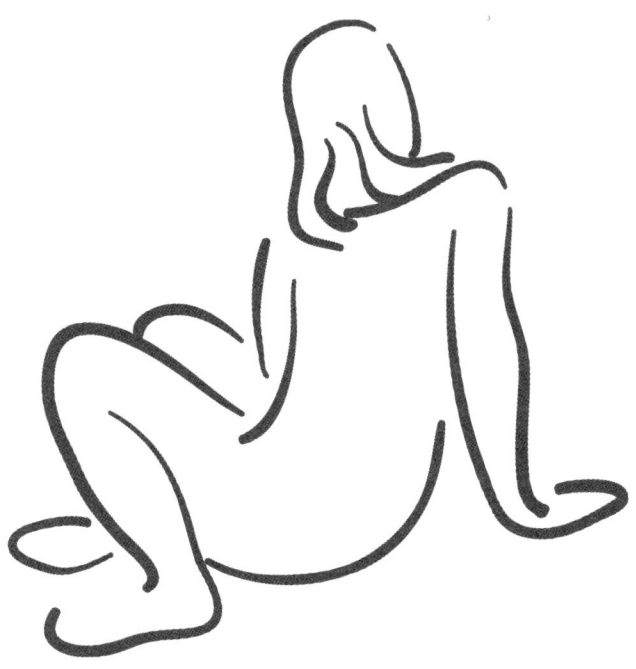

CHAPTER 1

An Ideal Body Image

Journal Entry

I felt so relaxed in Corpse Pose. As the image of my ideal body entered my thoughts I could feel the shift in my posture and the change in my sense of equilibrium. The muscles of my abdomen and scalp tightened.

I once came across a magazine feature article called "How to Change Your Self-Image in Five Easy Steps." The steps seemed logical and easy on the surface. But I thought it was sort of like telling someone how easy it would be to transplant a 5-foot tree in her yard. Those instructions could be made simple, too: You dig a hole, put your arms around the tree, pull it up by its roots, and move it over to the new spot. Articles like the one I read can be misleading because they ignore how deep and tenacious the roots of self-image are. For most of us five easy steps just won't be enough.

Changing a less-than-desirable self-image that results when you don't live up to the ideal image of how you want to look involves a significant personal transformation. Transformation, no matter how much you want a result, is generally not much fun. A friend summed it up succinctly when he said, "I want to be different, but I don't want to change."

Author William Bridges recognizes the difficulty of the transformation process in his book *Managing Transitions*. While Mr. Bridges' book focuses on transformation in business, his principles apply to any transformation. He says companies that implement changes in the workplace often fall way short of their optimistic goals because they overlook the significant personal adjustment employees must go through to effectively work with the new routines.

He metaphorically likens transformation to Moses' leading the Israelites out of Egypt. Egypt is the place where you live, but you are unhappy because it is limiting and you are not treated well there. The Promised Land is the dream of a better place where you want to go. But in order to get to the Promised Land, you need to go through the wilderness. The wilderness, which the author labels the "neutral zone," is a metaphor for transformation.

The wilderness of transformation can be a dark and scary place. Most of the time people stumble into it in spite of their best efforts to stay out. Few guideposts exist in the wilderness and one may have to wander around in confusion for periods of time. However, with the right kind of attitude and motivation, this untamed land is not only challenging, but also rewarding, offering many opportunities for new insights and breakthrough experiences.

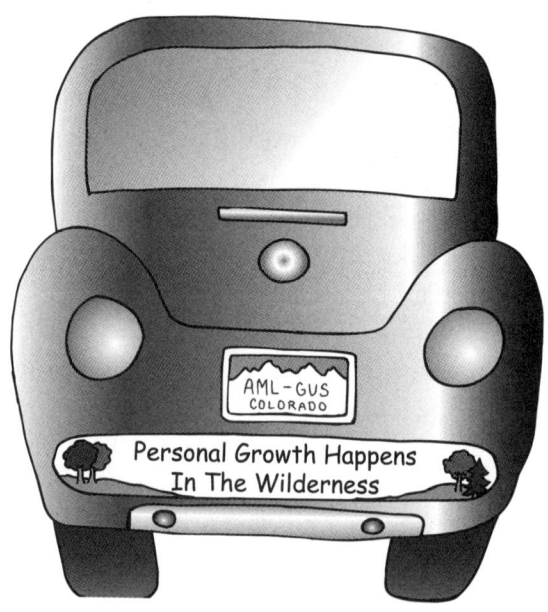

Corpse Pose Exercise

Try the following exercise, which uses a fundamental pose of yoga called the *Corpse Pose*, a pose of relaxation and total awareness. Play some soft background music, if you like.

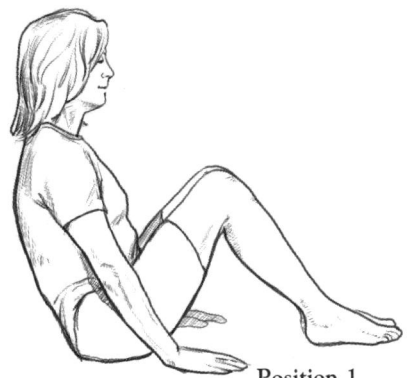

1. Sit on a carpeted floor with your knees bent.

2. Keeping your knees bent, roll your torso down, one vertebra at a time, until it is completely on the floor (see position 1).

Position 1

3. Relax your shoulders.

4. Relax your hips and thighs.

5. Lengthen and stretch out your right leg completely on the floor. Do the same with your left leg. Bring your arms out at a 45-degree angle, palms up.

6. Close your eyes by slowly lowering the top lid down to meet the bottom lid (see position 2).

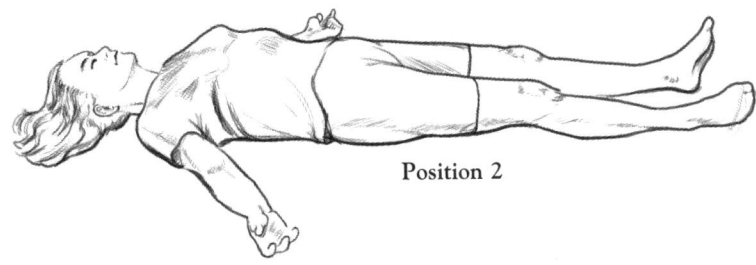

Position 2

7. Breathe deeply and slowly for five minutes. Let your breath become calmer, gentler, and softer, so your whole body becomes even more deeply relaxed.

8. Sink into the floor, feeling its support beneath you.

9. Corpse Pose looks and feels very comfortable and you may even fall asleep or space out, so try to keep yourself focused, alert, and aware of yourself and your surroundings.

10. When you feel very relaxed, continue.

11

11. Imagine that with each inhale you are feeling still more relaxed and lighter. Each breath makes you feel lighter and softer until you find yourself floating in a cloudless sky. The air is the same temperature as your skin.

12. Think of a place or an activity you enjoy, one that is peaceful and relaxing to you. For several minutes picture yourself in that place or doing that activity. Breathe in this scene until it fills every pore in your body. Notice how your body feels when you do this. Be aware of your body's posture, the expression on your face in this serene setting.

13. Let go of this image. Go back to floating in the sky again.

14. Now picture the ideal body image you visualized in the beginning exercise of this book. Notice if your mood and body change. Does your breathing change? Do you notice any change in the alignment and feel of your body that is different from the feeling of peace and tranquility?

15. If visualizing this body image disrupts your serenity in any way, inhale deeply and exhale any tension or anxiety. As you keep this image in mind, consciously bring your mood back to the feeling of peace and tranquility engendered by the serene setting with which you started the exercise. Focusing on breathing evenly and deeply throughout will help create the shift back. Does changing your breathing affect your reaction to your ideal image in any way?

16. Open your eyes and sit up.

This exercise should give you an opportunity to notice and reflect on how a thought pattern creates a physical response within your body. Habitual thoughts, of which the ideal body image is one, affect your body's equilibrium over a long period of time. The next time you feel anxious about your body's shape, see if you can remember to breathe deeply and relax, letting the anxiety go, just as you did in this exercise.

Write about your experience.

Part 2

Into the Wilderness

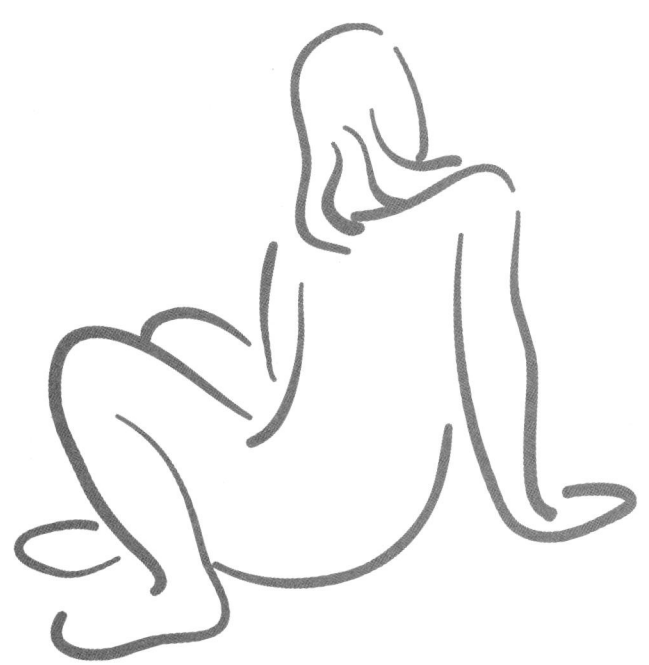

CHAPTER 2

Struggling With an Ideal Image

Up until that summer day I had always behaved as if my ideal image was a given. The problem had always been the unfortunate shape of my body. From that day on I made a firm decision to change this relationship with my body. I entered the wilderness resolutely.

I began by devising exercises for myself based on bits and pieces from self-help books and seminars. (My husband Bob attended the seminars; I just listened to what he had learned when he returned from them.)

I intensified my practice of yoga, eventually including qi gong—pronounced "chee gong," it means "energy work"—practiced by millions of Chinese. Both practices were the navigational instruments that guided me through the wilderness of transformation. They taught me the daily discipline that cultivates the formation of new habits and ideas. While the tennis experience was revealing, the practice of these disciplines, working with the whole of me—my mind, body, emotions, and spirit—was the force underlying my complete change of heart.

Journal Entry

Len, my former career counselor, taught me how to use timed writings. You start with a sentence and continue to write for ten minutes (or whatever time you set). You do not take your pencil off the paper, you just keep writing. If you get stuck, you write the word "stuck" until you think of something else to write. Or you can begin again with the first sentence. As you write without stopping, you often blurt out on the paper associations you are not consciously aware of. In this way, it brings subconscious thoughts to light.

Today I tried a timed writing about my stomach. I wrote "I hate my stomach because" and then continued writing, without stopping, for ten minutes. The object is to write, no matter what, for the full ten minutes. That wasn't hard at all.

When the timed writing was complete, I next tried the exercise starting with the opposite sentence, "I love my stomach because."

When I looked at what I had written, I noticed I started the first timed writing with physical traits. "I hate my stomach because it is hard, ugly, and too big." Midway through the writing I segued to character traits. "I hate my stomach because it is stubborn, rigid, and unyielding." Likewise with the "I love my stomach" part. I started with, "It digests food for me" and went on to "It is strong, willful, tenacious, a worthy adversary."

I substituted "myself " for "my stomach" and "I" for "it." The sentences became "I hate myself because I am stubborn and rigid." And, "I love myself because I am strong willed and tenacious." The revisions fit. A slightly more accurate tone to the statements would be "I hate myself when I am stubborn and rigid" and "I love myself when I am strong willed and tenacious."

My strong will and tenacity become stubbornness and rigidity when I am afraid.

I don't know why I direct my anger at myself toward my stomach. I guess one needs someplace to express the feeling. This tendency may be similar to the way one gets angry with a clerk who makes a mistake at the checkout counter of the grocery store when one is really angry with one's husband, or son, or father— or one's self.

A TV news program once reported on a survey that determined 49 percent of American women were displeased with some aspect of their bodies. A second TV news program quoted a different survey that reported a much higher percentage of 90 percent. My personal experience tells me this statistic might even be higher—more like 99.9 percent. I am sure she exists, but I don't know one woman who is completely comfortable with her body.

The most attractive women and the most accomplished women I know feel vulnerable about their looks. When I was an electrologist, I saw hundreds of female clients (from whom I probably removed billions and billions of unwanted body hairs), over the fourteen years I practiced the art. Every client with whom I ever had a personal conversation about personal appearance had an issue with some part of her body she didn't like.

Lynn, one of my best friends, is my age and an attractive, athletic woman. She has noted, and I tend to agree with her, that women who work out the most, who resemble the models in the magazines more than the rest of us, are often the most critical of their bodies.

My friend is an example of her own observation. Having lunch with her one day, I complimented her on her appearance since she resumed weight training. Her arms and chest looked toned and healthy. She was pleased with my compliment. However, she was still not satisfied with her looks because of her legs. I couldn't see her legs because she was wearing pants. I may have seen her legs maybe twice in the eighteen years of our friendship. On those two occasions they looked fine to me.

We had played out the rest of this conversation many times before. We gave each other mutual support. I reassured Lynn that she looked great, which she did. And she reassured me that I looked great. Because, of course, Lynn has always thought my stomach looks fine. It is probably not a candidate for Victoria's Secret lingerie ads, but to her it looks normal enough. She is my friend, not a modeling agent.

During our conversation at this lunch I was most struck by her tone, by the disdain I heard in her voice when she talked about her legs. Her emotional intensity, besides reminding me of myself, also reminded me of Maggie, another leg-hating friend of mine.

During her visit to Denver last summer, Maggie and I debated whether or not the media is responsible for the trouble we have with our self-images. She said, "Magazines like *Cosmopolitan* are at fault for the way we feel about ourselves." Curious to see what would happen, I asked her to try the timed writing exercise using her feelings about her legs.

I set a timer for ten minutes and she began the exercise with "I hate my legs because." When she was finished, I reset the timer for ten minutes and she began the second one with "I love my legs because (fill in the blank)."

For the first timed writing she wrote that she hated her legs because they were slow, heavy, plodding. For the second one, even though her pencil moved diligently for the full ten minutes, she didn't have much to say. "I need more time for that one," she said, "maybe twenty minutes." She grew pensive. "Maybe longer."

When we looked at what she had written, we noticed she hadn't mentioned *Cosmopolitan* once.

Soon after—and I don't think it was a coincidence—the subject of her relationship with her sister came up. She became glum and brooding as she said, "I have always felt inferior to my sister, like I am forever running to catch up with her, and I never do."

"What part of your anatomy do you run with?" I asked. She laughed.

Timed Writing Exercises

You will need a timer, pen or pencil, writing paper and a quiet place where you will not be disturbed. Choose the body part you dislike the most, if "hate" is not the right word or too strong, choose a more suitable one—choose the word or words you use most often when describing how you feel about this body part.

1. Set the timer for 10 minutes and begin with "I hate (or whatever other word you chose) my (fill in the blank with the body part) because (fill in the blank)."

2. Finish the sentence and then continue writing for the entire time. If you run out of things to say, you can write the word "stuck" until you are not stuck anymore. Or you can begin again with the original sentence "I (fill in the blank) my (fill in the blank) because (fill in the blank)."

3. Reset the timer for ten minutes and choose a word that is opposite in meaning to the word you picked for the first exercise.

4. Using the same body part, begin the second timed writing with a sentence using this second word. For example, if you chose "hate" then substitute "love," and so forth. "I love my (fill in the blank with the same body part you used in step 1) because (fill in the blank)."

5. Finish the sentence and then continue writing for the entire time, following the rules of step 2.

6. Try substituting "I" in the writings for the body part. For example, when my friend Maggie wrote, "I hate (my legs) because (they are plodding)," her substitute would be "I hate (myself) because (I am plodding)."

7. To take this substitution one step farther, change "because" to "when." My friend's final sentence reads "I hate myself *when* I am plodding."

After you have made the substitution ask yourself, "Is this a true statement about how I feel?" If so, ask yourself, "Are there specific times, specific people, or specific things I am doing when I am most likely to feel this way about myself?"

You can do this exercise several times over the course of several days. I find that if you ruminate on what you have written, it often reveals information similar to the kind you get when you keep a dream journal. The hints and clues to your subconscious thoughts are often metaphoric and symbolic, ones you can piece together, like a jigsaw puzzle, to reveal the bigger picture.

Also, take note of what you think about shortly after the exercise; for my friend Maggie, some of the connection was revealed later on.

Here are some other possible ways to start a timed writing:

"Because my (fill in the blank) are too fat, too small, too big, I am (fill in the blank)." Then do the opposite: "If my (fill in the blank) were thinner, larger, smaller, and so forth, I would be (fill in the blank)."

Or, "I can't let go of the image of how I want to look because (fill in the blank)."

Try other variations. Make up your own starting sentence and then do its opposite. Write for longer than ten minutes.

Timed Writings

Journal Entry

Stored within my consciousness, like an aged photograph, is a mental picture of myself standing next to my Aunt Jaye. We are in the living room of the Bronx apartment of my childhood. My aunt had taken me shopping and had bought me a dress in a style that was exactly like hers. The dress we are both wearing is a paisley print, with a blouse and a gathered skirt.

Underneath the elasticized waist of her dress, my aunt's stomach is perfectly flat. My young, 10-year-old self is training a perplexed eye on my own stomach, mildly unhappy with its shape, wishing it looked flatter. I can sense my 10-year-old stomach as round but soft. Over the years, both my stomach and attitude have hardened.

I focused on this picture of my younger self and breathed deeply and evenly. What was this 10-year-old girl feeling? She felt trapped.

I did a timed writing, starting with "I feel trapped when (fill in the blank)."

In the timed writing I recalled that my mother never let me abandon myself to a fun experience. I loved to jump rope. Only I would have to come inside before the other kids because she said I got "overheated." The next time out I would jump rope harder and faster to make up for what I would miss when I was made to come in. This meant I had to come in sooner because I got overheated more quickly.

As an adult I have rarely allowed myself to let go, to really have fun. When I schedule a "have fun, let go" experience, I get a headache from the effort. When I was young, my mother restricted me; now I restrict myself. Did I learn to be like my mother in this respect? Or was I really like her all along?

An English teacher once explained that fiction is made up of plot and theme. The plot is the action that occurs during the story, and the theme is what colors the action and gives it meaning. Theme explains why I can read murder mystery after murder mystery without getting bored. Even though the plots are essentially the same—someone gets murdered and you have to figure out who did it—the lives of the characters that unfold within the pages of these books create the interest.

The basic plot of life is simple—we are born, grow up, and die. The themes of life are what give these events their unique meanings. The themes are filled with our emotions—our expectations and fears, our feelings of failure or success, joy or sadness, guilt, vindication.

And so much of who we are and what we experience in the present is based on our memories of who we were and what we experienced in the past.

Margaret—my sister—and I once argued over which one of us received more favored treatment from our aunts.

"You did," she said. "Aunt Jaye used to polish your nails and wouldn't touch mine because I bit them."

I don't remember that. What I do remember was that our Aunt Ann would always polish my sister's nails first, which made me feel like I was second-best. That, Margaret doesn't remember.

Do my sister and I have a slighted past or do we have a past of remembered slights? The mental picture I carry around of Aunt Jaye and me, dressed in our paisley dresses, is powerful because it evokes emotions that are still present, just as the feeling of being somehow permanently slighted still lingers. "I don't get what I want," is a familiar refrain. I can feel my diaphragm tighten as I repeat the phrase.

Memory connects us to our emotional past. In his work with the clients he counsels, my husband Bob describes emotions as being charged, like magnets. The positive and negative pulls from our emotionally charged memories reach out into the events we experience in the present, affecting our current behavior. To describe an event as emotionally charged has more meaning in this context.

In one of her classes, my astrologer gave a humorous example of how this magnetic charge works. She depicted a scenario in which a man and a woman meet at a party. As their eyes find each other across the room, they both feel a jolt, like an electric current; they are instantly aware of a strong attraction to each other. This setting is pretty romantic, a great scene for a novel.

However, to make her point about magnetic charges, my astrologer envisions a different, not-so-romantic scenario taking place on the subconscious level. Our heroine, who needs to learn how to accept her own worthiness in a relationship, repeatedly gets abandoned. Her love interest, who needs to learn how to be comfortable with intimacy, repeatedly abandons the people he dates. A perfect fit. The electrical circuit of attraction is complete.

Try the following memory exercises.

Memory Exercises

1. Sit comfortably on a chair with your feet resting on the floor and parallel to each other. Straighten your spine and rest your hands lightly on your thighs.

2. Breathe evenly through both nostrils.

3. Deepen your breath, direct it down into your abdomen and then fill up your chest. Make the inhalations equal to the exhalations.

4. Close your eyes.

5. Visualize the first time you were uncomfortable with what you dislike most about your body. Make the memory as clear and as detailed as possible. Take your time. Do you remember how old you were, where you were, what you were wearing, who you were with? Do any sights, sounds, or smells come back to you?

6. Breathe deeply for several minutes, as you stay focused on this memory.

7. Can you remember an earlier time in your life when you felt this same discomfort? If so, explore this memory as you did the first one. How old were you? What were you doing? Who were you with?

8. Next, see if an even earlier memory comes to mind. Keep going until you exhaust your ability to remember any farther back. In this earliest memory, what were you feeling? What were you thinking? What did you need? Did you need to be hugged or held? Did you need to be left alone? Have you given what you needed to yourself? Can you give it now? If so, do so.

9. Keeping this earliest scenario in mind, say to yourself "I cannot remember (fill in the blank)" and see if anything else comes into your picture.

10. Open your eyes.

Write about your experience in the space provided. Try a timed writing with the feelings you experienced. Start with I feel (whatever the feeling was) when I (fill in the blank). Then try a timed writing substituting the opposite feeling.

Here's a second exercise to try:

If you visualized anyone in your memory sequence, set up an imaginary dialogue with that person, ask him or her any questions you would like, say anything you would like.

What feelings from this past memory are still present now? Select one that surfaced. Focus on this emotion and notice the changes that take place in your posture, your breathing, your sense of well-being. Can you create the opposite emotion within you?

And a third:

Try accessing a different memory every day for a week and see how far back in time you can go. Write about each experience. Then compare and see if any significant patterns emerge.

Memory Notes

.

Journal Entry

> *"Work on the body parts we hate," exhorted the author of a book I came across in the bookstore. I have worked on the body part I hate and my feelings about it haven't changed. Exercise cannot fix what is wrong with it.*
>
> *I observed my reaction to the pictures of flat-stomached models in the magazines at the grocery store checkout counter. These pictures evoked a familiar mosaic of thoughts and emotions: despair that my stomach was too big and too round, resolve that I would work very hard to fix it, and earnest, euphoric optimism that what I wanted was feasible.*
>
> *In recent years it seems a more busty look has gained prominence as a feature of fitness ads. Yet I have never wanted larger breasts, even though by the standards of these ads, I could sure use some help. Nor have I ever wanted "buns of steel." Sound bites are effective when one is vulnerable, yet can be funny when one is not. Whenever I see ads for buns of steel I picture a butt made of two Brillo pads, scrubbing against each other as one walks. I'll keep my softer, spongier buns, thank you.*

Most workouts in the gym, while very beneficial and healthy, usually do nothing to address the pain that results in a lack of a healthy sense of self. Sometimes it seems the more we work out, the more we buy into the ideal image.

If it is true that we hate parts of our body because they do not match the standards of beauty created by the media, then why are we okay with some areas of our bodies that do not conform to the images we see in magazines and on TV?

My experience says that the status of our self-confidence is reflected in our mind/body connection. Where we are confident and our mind/body connection is strong and balanced, we have a sense of well-being and a strong sense of self. Where we are less sure of ourselves, where the connection is not strong or balanced, we don't. In those areas we look outside of ourselves for cues. And the media is definitely good at supplying us with cues.

Thought Exercises

Exercise 1

Are you happy with parts of your body that do not conform to conventional standards of beauty? Why do you like them anyway?

Try a timed writing with I love my (insert a body part you are happy with) because (fill in the blank).

Exercise 2

1. Sit comfortably on a chair with both feet resting on the floor.

2. Close your eyes and breathe deeply and evenly for two minutes.

3. Focus your attention on the body part in the first exercise. Notice how you feel when you do.

4. Focus your attention on a body part you dislike and notice how your feeling changes.

5. What does your body part in exercise 1 have to say to the body part you dislike?

6. What response does the body part you dislike make?

7. Continue the dialogue with whatever comes to mind.

8. When the dialogue runs out, and if you haven't already, ask the body part you like if there is anything it can do to help out the body part you dislike.

Workbook Space

Journal Entry

    I don't think you can predict by looking at her which part of her body a woman feels most vulnerable about. Nicki, my friend for more than twenty years—one of the brightest, most accomplished people I know—recently shocked me when she confessed she has always felt that her nose is too big. In all of the years I have known her I have never thought of her nose as anything but well, normal. She has always wanted to be taller, too. She has become taller in a way—she has great stature in her chosen field of psychotherapy. Being a therapist, the connection between her desire to be tall and her "tall" professional stature is not lost on her.

    Every woman I know seems to dislike something about her body. One of my friends hates her thin hair, another hates her heavy thighs and my former tennis partner hates her fat knees.

    Fat knees—that's a new one to me. I've never thought of knees as fat or skinny. To me, they are simply ugly by nature and are best hidden under pants or a long dress—legs look better without them.

    I asked my friend Nicki if she had ever heard of fat knees.

    She most certainly had—one of her friends has fat knees to prove it.

    I talked to my friend Annuradha today. She asked how my body project was coming along. "Don't we all wish we had Christy Brinkley thighs," she sighed. I have no idea what Christy Brinkley's thighs look like. I don't usually notice thighs.

    I did notice my thighs for a while, though. For a very short time I controlled my eating enough to get a flat stomach. Family and friends told me I was too thin. I didn't think so. With my stomach flat, I began to notice how fat my thighs looked. When I went back to a more normal weight my stomach rounded out and I forgot about my fat thighs.

Have you ever "fixed" one part of your body and then discovered another part that didn't measure up? A part that hadn't bothered you before? Or have you ever been as surprised as I was that a friend hated a part of her body you thought was perfectly normal?

31

CHAPTER 3

Discovering Yoga

As I wrote in my journal and worked with my visualizations and timed exercises, I continued my daily practice of yoga for an hour or more each day.

I had first considered taking up yoga to become more flexible when my husband Bob started taking classes at his gym. I was then thirty-seven, with an increasing sense that my lack of flexibility was a problem I needed to address. As young as my early twenties I could barely reach my fingers to the middle of my shins when I bent over. I wasn't concerned at the time. I regarded my lack of flexibility as an intrinsic characteristic, like the shape of my nose.

My attitude started to change when my son Neill was born and I was thirty-three years old. After my pregnancy I returned to the gym to resume aerobic and weight training. A young fitness trainer tested me for reentry back into the gym. She noted on my chart that my strength was fine. However, she graded my flexibility to be in the danger zone. "Flunking" the flexibility test did not surprise me, but the obvious concern in her voice and the "danger zone" connotation scared me a little.

Several years later, when Bob started taking yoga classes to become more flexible, I thought about the same possibility for myself. Not one to rush into things, I attended my first class five years after him.

Serendipity brought me Isabelle, my first yoga teacher. Shopping in a local health market one day, I stepped on a flyer advertising yoga classes in her home. I called her that day and arranged to attend her next class.

The leg extensions of my first yoga class were the most memorable of the poses. Lying supine on the floor, a student bends the knee of one leg, resting the foot on the floor. She then loops a strap around the foot of the other leg, brings it toward her chest and extends it—theoretically—straight up into the air toward the ceiling.

I followed the directions as best I could. The grinding pain I felt when I extended my leg into the air was that of trying to force a rusted machine to move without oiling it first. It never made it past a 90-degree bend. And it shook and wobbled the whole time it was extended. Isabelle later confided that seeing how painfully stiff I was, she hadn't expected me to return after that first class. Fortunately I did. People like me need yoga the most.

I not only attended class each week but also practiced daily at home. One memorable day, two months into my practice, my tenacity was rewarded. My body began to vibrate on its own after a session of yoga. It vibrated for hours with the release of

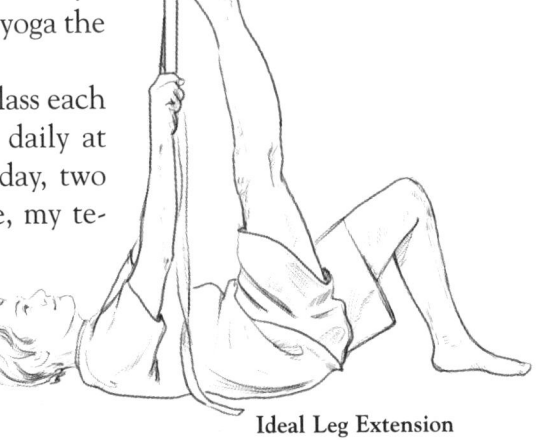

Ideal Leg Extension

wave after wave of stored tension, bringing tremendous physical relief. I felt as if an invisible masseuse with magical fingers had been set to work on me. Afterward I was limp but happy.

The physical relief from the release of oceans of stored tension was the greatest reward of those first few months of my practice. It would take a while, however, for the lessons learned in my practice to begin to noticeably alter the chronic anxiety I felt about my body's shape.

Yoga teaches you to be patient and tolerant with your body. But in the beginning I looked in yoga books and magazines and saw people in postures I could only dream of doing. I revised my ideal body image accordingly.

Updated ideal body image: Julie Christie's nose, a 21-inch waist, a stomach in line with the front tips of my hipbone—in Wheel pose.

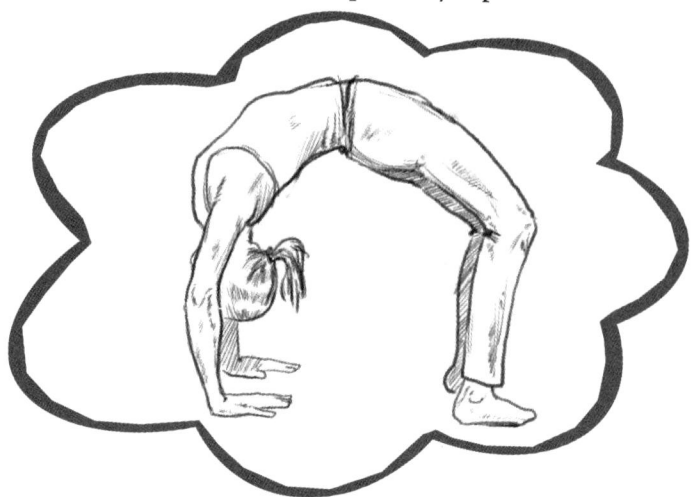

Sometimes things get worse before they get better.

Journal Entry

Huge stomach attack!

When I woke up this morning, my stomach was its normal round self. I had a bowl of cereal and went into my room to work. Work did not go well. By midmorning my stomach felt huge. I am amazed; it is like a shape-shifter, turning huge in the blink of an eye. How can it transform itself from normal to huge in two hours?

I looked at my profile in the mirror. If I stretched myself tall, my stomach became smaller. If I slouched and exaggerated my usual sway back posture it seemed bigger. If I stood normal straight, its size was somewhere in between the two extremes. My stomach, waist and hips didn't look too bad if I isolated them from the rest of my body. However, if I compared the upper and lower halves of my torso, the lower half seemed too wide and bulky. I was confused. Out of the corner of my eye, reality was shifting from one possibility to another.

Lynn called. I told her about my stomach. She said, "Barbara, your stomach gets bigger after you have eaten." What she said is true. But I don't think that small bowl of cereal could account for the exaggerated feeling of hugeness. Internally, the hugeness felt infinitely big. Its vastness felt like the expanding stomachs in those TV ads for antacid. Only I didn't have indigestion.

When I told Lynn about my confusion examining my body in the mirror she understood exactly what I meant. She also gets confused sometimes looking at her body in the mirror.

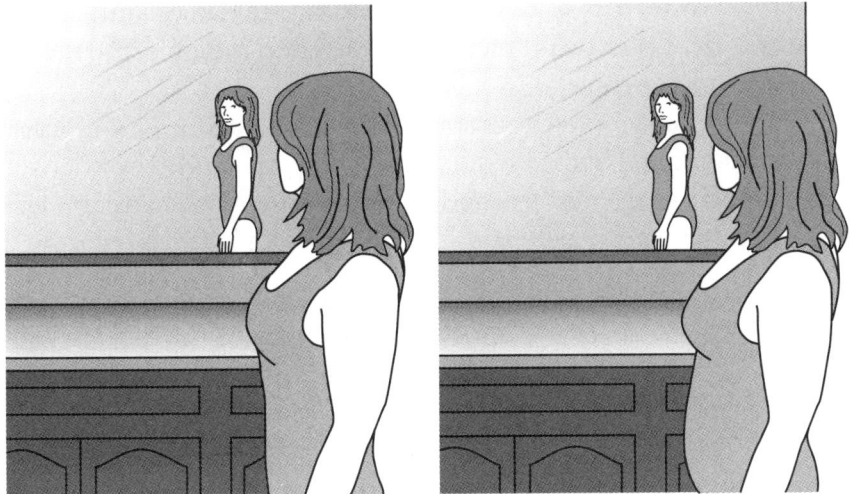

Why do we, living, three-dimensional people, use our two-dimensional reflections in the mirror to compare and measure ourselves? I don't think we do ourselves justice as women when we do this. We compare and measure our two-dimensional images to the lifeless, two-dimensional images of people we see in magazines, books, and on TV. We focus on the surface shape of our bodies, treating ourselves as objects.

Bridget Jones's Diary by Helen Fielding is a frank and funny chronicle of one year in the life of a young, single woman named Bridget. At one point in the book Bridget contemplates developing "inner poise" to help her feel better about her body and herself. The thought is a fleeting one, sandwiched between her ongoing struggle to lose weight, quit smoking, and find love.

The Random House Dictionary carries the following definition for poise: "a state of balance or equilibrium, stability." The development of inner poise is a good way to describe the kind of change that takes place internally and enables you to see yourself more positively when you practice yoga. The sense of balance and equilibrium you cultivate in yoga poses prepares you to look past surface features and be comfortable with the "real" person inside. This sense of balance and equilibrium, this inner poise comes from a harmonious blend of the mind, emotions, body, and spirit.

Inner poise is not possible when you make yourself an object. It comes from exploring the inner shape of your body. With the cultivation of inner poise you are less likely to make unhealthy comparisons of your two-dimensional reflection in a mirror to media images or other people.

The following exercise comes from my Phoenix Rising Yoga Therapy training. Phoenix Rising Yoga Therapy, founded by Michael Lee, combines yoga postures and dialogue to help you better understand the connection between your thoughts and your body.

Inner/Outer Exercise

1. Stand in front of a mirror.

2. Relax and breathe naturally for five minutes.

3. Focus on your breath as it enters and leaves your body. Observe its rhythm without altering it.

4. Now breathe more slowly and deeply. Let your breath reach down into and fill up your lower abdomen. Make the inhalation and the exhalation of equal length. Do this for another five minutes.

5. Soften your gaze by imagining that your eyes are located at the back of your head. Look out into the world with your gaze coming forward from the back of your head.

   Notice how focusing your gaze in this way relaxes your eyes. Explore the inner shape of your body as follows:

6. Close your eyes by bringing your upper lid down to meet your lower lid.

7. Focus your attention on your right foot. Imagine your breath traveling all the way down to the sole of your foot. Focus your attention inside of your foot. Is it relaxed or tense? Is the space inside of your foot light or dark? Do you feel happy or sad there?

What are the boundaries of the space inside of your foot? Can you tell if the inner space extends to fill out each toe? Each heel? Your instep? Or are there areas within your foot that seem closed off to you?

Move your attention up to your right ankle. Explore its inner space in the same manner. Move up your leg, exploring inside your lower leg, knee, and thigh.

Starting at your left foot, do the same exploration of your left leg.

8. Continue up to your hips, solar plexus, chest, arms, neck, and head. End at the crown of your head. Take your time and explore every nook and cranny. Also notice if you experience any sights, smells, or sounds anywhere.

9. When you have reached the crown of your head, blend all the areas of your body into one another and feel your inner shape as a whole.

10. Open your eyes. Again look out from the back of your head, this time with the awareness of the inner shape you just explored. Gaze at the outer form you see in the mirror with this awareness.

With inner poise you observe yourself from the center of your being.

Journal Entry

While in my car on the way to the grocery store, I noticed how my arm was draped protectively over my abdomen. I was hiding it from view as I squirmed in discomfort. Another fat stomach day. Took some deep breaths, trying to dispel some of the emotional heaviness I felt inside. My struggle with my body's shape felt like a burden, a ball and chain that I drag along with me everywhere.

"Why does this burden follow me? Why doesn't it just go away?" I silently agonized. I mentally pictured the ball and chain, working my vision down to the end of the attachment, which was at my ankles. I am struggling against myself. While I am trying to pry myself free of the chain with one hand, I am gripping it tightly, holding on for dear life, with the other hand.

Ah, as a famous Shakespearean character says, "Therein lies the rub." I heard an inner voice, like a mental tap on the shoulder whispering, "Psst, you dummy, all you have to do is let it go."

When Neill was little, I wanted to be a perfect parent. I knew I wasn't perfect, I even accepted the fact that there probably was no such thing as a perfect parent. However, some naughty little voice would whisper inside my head that if a perfect parent existed, it would have to be someone who could admit she wasn't perfect.

This is Catch-22 thinking. I am still playing mind games. I am hoping that if I love and accept myself as I am, my body will magically turn into the Julie Christie/Barbie doll image of how I have wanted to look all along. Sort of a cosmic reward for being good.

Remember the ideal body image exercise on page 4? Were you able to visualize how you are attached to your ideal image? Use that vision now for the following exercise or take this opportunity to try the visualization again:

Attachment Exercises

Exercise 1

1. Close your eyes and take a few deep breaths.

2. Visualize your attachment to your image. Maybe you see the same attachment as you did in the previous exercise. Maybe you don't. Either case is fine.

3. Visualize what it would take for you to let go of your attachment. Can you comfortably see yourself letting it go or do you experience feelings of anxiety or fear when you contemplate the prospect?

Exercise 2

Try a timed writing: "I am attached to my image by (fill in the blank)."

Exercise 3

Every morning for one week, first thing when you wake up, ask yourself what you can do during the day to loosen or even release yourself from the attachment. Do whatever comes to mind first, if at all possible.

Attachment Notes

Journal Entry

Last night's dream—I am seated on a hillside cuddled in one of my yoga blankets. The sky beyond is a brilliant kaleidoscope in hues of blue and red and green. As I gaze at it, as if on some cue, the sky turns gray. Its shifting geometric patterns coalesce into a raging, windy vortex in front of me. The vortex is so powerful that I am terrified of being swept away. My arms cross protectively over my chest as I dig in to resist.

End of dream.

I knew intuitively that the vortex embodies the emotional turmoil created by my attachment to the way things should be. Were I willing to let go of the attachment, the turmoil—and therefore the vortex—would disappear. If I want to end the struggle with my body, I have to surrender the image of how I want it to look.

But I don't want to surrender.

Letting go of some attachments is very hard, however if your desire is strong enough you will find the way to do it.

After two years with Isabelle, I started to take classes with Debra Ann, my present yoga teacher.

Journal Entry

"Let go, let go, let go." For the past four-plus years, over and over again, those are Debra Ann's instructions in class. Today we did Cobbler's Pose lined up with our backs against the wall. My legs formed a narrow "V" in the pose. I looked around the class and saw the most flexible student stretch out until almost the entire length of her thighs was resting on the floor. I tried to force my knees down but they wouldn't move no matter how much effort I focused on them. They just wouldn't budge.

Debra Ann came over to me. "Relax and let go in the groin," she said. I Cobbler's Pose: Cobblers in India put the shoes in between their feet as they work.

shifted my focus away from my knees. My mind searched my
groin for a sense of awareness, but couldn't find any. Yet I knew
it was there because it hurt.

One of my friends is avoiding yoga because she is so stiff. I don't
blame her; a stiff body feels a lot of pain in yoga classes for a while. In
his book *Bikram's Beginning Yoga*, Bikram Choudhury describes the
process of yoga as "waking up the body." Sometimes a resurrection
from the dead seems more in order.

Waking up your body, or resurrecting it, as the case may be, can
be uncomfortable for a while, but it is worth the effort. Your body
becomes stronger, more flexible, healthier. So does your mind. Yoga
wakes up your body and your mind; you begin to peer into corners of
both that you may have kept roped off for years. You wake up emotions you may have wanted to keep buried in these corners forever.

The training you get through yoga practice develops the courage
you need to face the closed off areas in your body and in your life,
the courage you need to let go of an idealistic/unrealistic body image
and create the strong sense of self you desire. When you understand
how to access these closed off areas, these "dead zones," using a concept called "the edge," you will have a tool for creating this change.

Dead Zones

I love the psychological term "gestalt," which I learned from
Nicki. It means to grasp something as a unified whole, to understand
its essence as that whole something that is more than the sum of its
parts.

During lunch one day a friend ruefully proclaimed his feet to be
dead. He didn't have gangrene, or a fatal foot disease. For two years
he had been receiving massage and other bodywork from a woman
who used her own special blend of techniques. His gestalt, that his
feet were somehow dead, was the result of his gradual awakening to
the lack of their mind/body communication. One of the physical
results of this lack was immobile, painful, and disconnected feet.
Dead feet.

Tight, habitually contracted areas of the body are often so inaccessible to conscious awareness that they feel dead (like my friend's

feet and my groin). I call these areas dead zones. A dead zone is a place where the mind and body no longer communicate with one another and is the worst of two worlds. It is dead in the sense that it is cut off from communication and at the same time it is often very painful. While excessively stiff people like myself have such an overall lack of mobility it is easy for us to recognize dead zones, even some of the most flexible people I have known have dead zones.

For example, one of my friends who used to practice ballet has great flexibility in her lower body but very tight, sore areas in her upper body. Additionally, even the most flexible areas of a body are not necessarily hooked up to conscious awareness.

A person can be oblivious to some dead zones. Several years ago I visited an attorney to put my parents' estate in order. After finishing with the estate business we got on to other topics, and he asked me about my experiences in yoga. To demonstrate how tight, contracted muscles sap energy from the body, I asked him to tense the muscles of his left arm and hold them tight for as long as possible. The muscles of his upper arm obeyed his inner command but the muscles in his lower arm didn't respond. He was startled. He had been unaware of this lack of conscious communication. His perfectly normal-looking muscles were dead zones.

Discovering dead zones can be daunting. He ignored what had happened and immediately changed the subject.

The essence of dead zones reminds me of the experience I had driving Neill to work one summer. Whenever I go anywhere I take the major roads, never thinking about alternatives. As I started to take my usual route to his job one day, Neill guided me to a shortcut I had not known existed. As the summer progressed, he showed me four different routes, composed of quiet meandering neighborhood roads, to his summer job. Surprised, I asked him how he knew of all of these different routes. He replied that he and his friends had discovered them while driving through the neighborhood, with nothing else to do, on weekend evenings.

As I began to pay attention to them, I discovered other less-traveled roads in my neighborhood. One time I followed an Access-A-Ride bus that was bringing my father home from church. The driver took a shortcut that halved the driving time. The driver, out of necessity, and my son, out of idle time, found more options, more range of motion driving around in the neighborhood than I did. Their internal maps of the area were much more intricate than mine was.

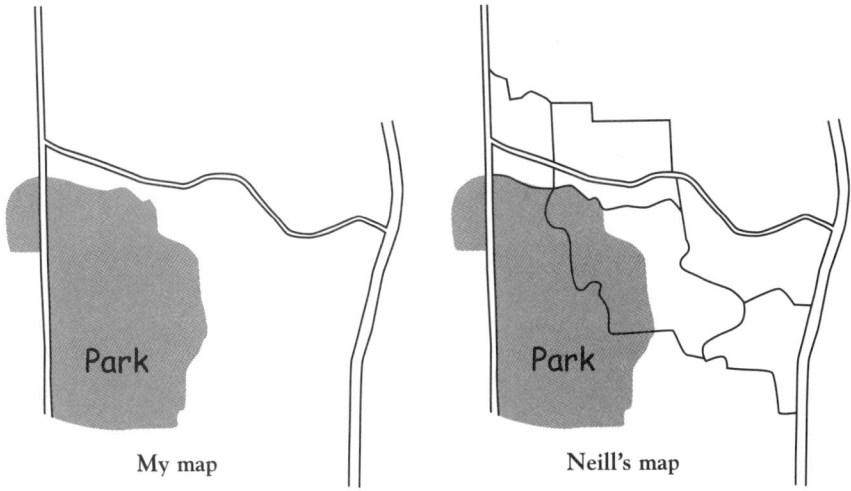

My map   Neill's map

Dead zones in the body are like these less-traveled roads. They are less-traveled roads in your body. You may have once had access to them when younger, but that was so long ago that you have forgotten about their existence. Dead zones limit your body's range of motion. They are unhealthy and they also change the shape of your body; they help to create the crooked postures of old age.

I learned about the term "range of motion" from the therapists who helped my mother after she was diagnosed with Parkinson's Disease. This term refers to your body's mobility—for example the ability of your head to turn from one side to the other, or the ability of your arms and legs to move in their sockets, or of your spine to bend and twist. As most of us age our range of motion decreases. Over time we narrow the available routes of movement in our body maps.

This decreasing ability to move is not an inevitable part of aging. A qi gong master, who lived to be 100 years old, is pictured at an advanced age on the cover of a book in the following posture.

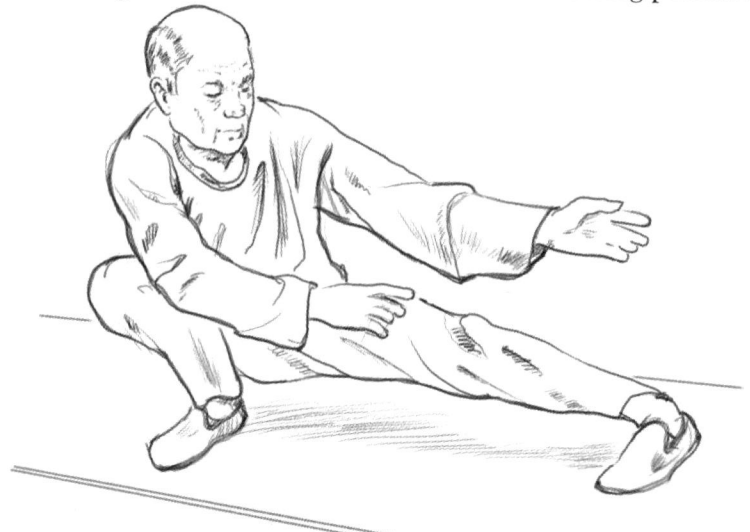

I would love to be as flexible as he is.

One of the rewarding aspects of life is that we learn from our mistakes and we build up a reservoir of knowledge to operate from. One of the limiting aspects of life is that we build up a reservoir of knowledge and stop looking for new possibilities.

When driving, I choose only the major roads out of expediency without giving thought to other options. This mirrors the way I approach many aspects of my life. I think many of us narrow our options in life all of the time. We repeatedly choose the same, comfortable routes out of habit. We construct a lifestyle in which we protect ourselves, one that concentrates on some areas of our lives but ignores others. This very normal tendency is reflected in our bodies. We also narrow our bodies' options of motion. As we age we lose the full range of motion we had when we were children. This process often proceeds along its course without our awareness, until eventually we feel old, tired, and stiff.

I practiced on friends for my Phoenix Rising Yoga Therapy training, guiding them into yoga postures and encouraging a flow of dialogue as they held the poses. I found they were often surprised by their lack of mobility in different areas of their bodies. They were not aware of how their bodies had changed over the years. For example, one forty-year-old friend trying to do Child's Pose (see picture) was surprised she was too stiff in her knees and hips to rest her buttocks on her heels. She remembered being able to easily

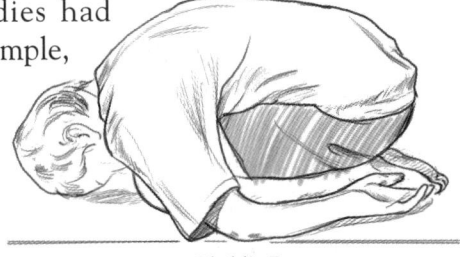

Child's Pose

sit this way when she was younger. Child's Pose brought the decrease in her range of motion to her attention.

Dead zones are unused pathways within our bodies that have become so overgrown with weeds that we forget where they are. We need to systematically search for them, to locate the edges of their boundaries so we can begin making inroads into the richness of their forgotten depths.

Finding the Edge: Locating and Making Inroads Into Dead Zones

Whenever I had a new client consultation in my electrolysis practice, I would tell her the procedure had a certain amount of discomfort. It hurt. Dead zones often hurt when you approach them. Much of the discomfort (i.e. pain) in yoga postures comes from a body that is not in balance, either from the stiffness and soreness of habitually contracted muscles or from the weakness of overextended areas. Every yoga teacher I have ever had has dealt with this problem. Michael Lee labeled the boundary of the discomfort "the edge."

In his book *Stretching*, Bob Anderson uses a similar concept, he breaks down a good stretch into these parts.

Easy Stretch	Developmental Stretch	Drastic Stretch
(Held for 20–30 seconds)	(Held for 30 seconds or longer)	(Avoid)

Referring to the picture, the edge in yoga would be comparable to the developmental part of stretching in the middle section. The edge is located along the outer boundaries where you no longer have conscious access to your body. A yoga pose guides you to the edge, which brings you as close as possible to the closed-off territories of your body. They are where you have inhibited your range of motion in your body and your mind, so you are not as flexible to move through life as you were when you were younger.

Daily practice with the edge teaches you how to safely enter these dead zones. You locate a thread of conscious awareness along the borders of a dead zone and work to expand from there. As you follow this thread it leads you deeper inside, creating open paths of awareness.

Very often the first response when you reach this edge is to tense and draw away. Sometimes the feeling is stronger; i.e., you want to get the hell out of there as quickly as possible. Yet as you stay within its territory and relax and stretch out with deep, expansive breathing, the discomfort recedes and you can move further into your dead zone.

The edge does not create pain. It unlocks and releases the pain already in your body. The edge is a three-dimensional, mental, emotional, physical plane where less effort is not enough to make any forward progress, and more effort is too much. Within the edge you can expand your physical, mental, and emotional boundaries without hurting yourself.

The edge is transformational; it is located in the wilderness.

Journal Entry

I once heard an "open mind" described as the ability to listen to and assimilate what you hear without immediately changing it into your own words. Without trying to fit it into your existing frame of reference. After all, how are you going to expand your frame of reference if everything is supposed to fit into the one you already have?

I wasn't sure if today was a fat stomach day or thin stomach day. I struggled with my view in the mirror, looked sideways, stretched myself up and down, but the results were inconclusive. On these borderline days when I just can't tell for sure if I am fat or not I let the scale settle the matter. One hundred and twelve pounds or under is thin, anything over that is fat.

One hundred thirteen pounds. A fat stomach day.

Felt adventurous. Jeans are thin stomach clothes. On some days, just to be different, I will wear the one pair I own. And it has to be on a day that my stomach is relatively thin.

Old framework: "I can't wear my jeans on a fat stomach day."

Open mind thought: "I can wear and be comfortable in jeans on a fat stomach day."

I squirmed with discomfort as I put on my jeans. I sucked in my solar plexus and stomach so hard I could barely breathe. Looked fat in the mirror. I almost always look fat in jeans, which is why I hardly ever wear them. I took deep breaths into my solar plexus and abdomen and stayed within the mental/emotional edge of my discomfort. The ideal body I aspired to, made a line that cut off part of my stomach. What was left outside of the line was fat and caused me pain.

Continued to breathe and focus on the sad, unhappy sensation of fatness as it surfaced. After a while the pain lessened. I envisioned a new line drawn around my abdominal area, one that eased the shape of my ideal image to fit around my real stomach. The mental/emotional edge softened. Felt better, more relaxed.

Wore the jeans for the whole day.

Felt good about my success with the challenge. In my heart I know I would have to be anorexic-thin in order to measure up to my ideal image.

I once watched a TV program about a treatment for people with agoraphobia (people who don't leave their house because of their fear of being in an open space). Part of their therapy consists of regular practice in conquering their fear and developing the ability to leave their house. Their edge in the therapy is to venture as far away from their house as they are able to each time that they leave it. One person shown on this program was only able to go as far as her door the first time she tried. Then after some additional forays she was able to walk down her driveway to her mailbox, and so on.

An ideal body image can be as mentally confining as a house you are physically afraid to venture out of. Beyond the confines of an ideal image is a wide open space of possible ways you could perceive your body to look, and still be happy with it. Your challenge is to leave the confined space of your image, to explore these alternatives. But you have to take a step toward this new vista, "to step outside of the house." Try the exercises at the end of this section more than once.

The edge of the experience in these exercises is to go the limit of your endurance without hurting yourself, and stay there until you get used to it. You'll find that the edge will change and you will go further out to a new edge. This is the personal growth aspect of it.

Edge Exercises

There is nothing wrong with wanting to look your best, to accentuate your best features when you dress. However, if you pick out clothes or wear makeup to disguise yourself, to try to change your body into something it isn't, this is the kind of behavior to address in this and the following exercises.

Decide on a day to change the way you dress or make yourself up, just to see what happens.

Exercise 1

Pick out the body part you dislike the most. Envision how you can challenge the feeling that its flaws are so awful that you have to disguise them. Maybe you can pick out something you would not wear because you are on the heavier side of your usual weight this day, or it is a "fat thigh, bad hair, big butt day," and so forth.

Think carefully, maybe the challenge is in your makeup, or something else you do to habitually disguise what you consider to be your worst flaws.

You will bring yourself to the edge of discomfort by behaving as differently as you can possibly imagine, by doing the opposite of what you would normally do.

If you aren't able to leave the house the first time you try this, practice inside of the house. If you cannot carry through with your plan, mentally picture yourself doing it. Write about the feelings that come up when you think about trying this exercise.

Whatever discomfort you experience, you can soften its impact by softening your mental/emotional edge. Revise the boundaries of how you think you should look to fit around the body you have.

Exercise 2

Every morning for at least one week ask yourself what you can do that day to heal your self-image. If it is feasible, do it. Try to make this an intuitive exercise, one where you just follow whatever first comes into your mind. Keep a journal of your experiences.

Develop other exercises that challenge your habitual patterns of behavior that are based upon an inability to accept your body/yourself.

Journal Entry

Made a discovery in qi gong standing meditation today. I explained to Zhu that if I relax my pelvis—more precisely the floor of my pelvis—where the perineum is, only inside, I am able for the first time to access and release some of the stiffness in the front of my ankles. Zhu nodded. He said, pointing to my pelvic area, "That is the root of the body. The feet and the head are the top."

Resisted the temptation to revise what Zhu had said to fit in with the biological view I already have. How can the feet be the top of the body if you stand on them? A mind that is open says not to judge it as right or wrong, nor to revise it in familiar language, but just accept it as a different view. In this way you broaden your perspective and learn what this new view has to teach you.

Zhu was viewing the body in terms of the flow of qi (energy).

Did Forward Bend using Bikram's Beginning Yoga book. Following his directions, you grab your big toes with your fingers and pull. I guess that sometimes pulling is okay in yoga postures. It just depends on what is happening in the pose when you do so. Bikram's technique keeps your body aligned so that the pulling forces you to relax where you are holding on. Your body is positioned in such a way that the pulling not only highlights but underlines, double, the tight areas.

I thought some open mind exercises might look like this:

Taking different routes home from work or to the grocery store.

Choosing the opposite side of an issue you feel strongly about and arguing from that point of view with passion.

Did an "opposite" experiment with my stomach. When I look in the mirror I am often confused about my stomach's size. Is it really too big? Since I can't step outside of myself to see, I have to rely on a two-dimensional reflection.

Closed my eyes and focused on my stomach. Imagined it getting larger and denser. Made it feel as large and as dense as possible.

When I reached the maximum, I released the sensations of heaviness and density. Then I imagined my stomach getting smaller and lighter. Made it smaller and lighter until I couldn't make it any more so. Then I released the sensations of smallness and lightness.

I sensed a midpoint between the two extremes, a neutral point of balance. My stomach felt "normal" for those few seconds. This normality came from an inner sense of balance, not from a reflection in my mirror.

(Note: Zhu is my qi gong teacher; I will describe the experience of qi gong in more detail later.)

Opposite Exercise

Try this exercise with a body part that doesn't measure up to your expectations.

1. Close your eyes and breathe deeply and evenly for several moments.

2. Focus your breath on the body part you don't like. To help direct your breath, place your hands on this area and breathe into the touch of your hands.

3. Exaggerate the undesirable trait of this body part. Coordinate the imagery with the flow of your breath. For example, if you have fat thighs, imagine them fatter with each inhale; keep going until you can't make them any fatter.

4. Let go of the sensation.

5. Remain focused on the body part and exaggerate the opposite quality. Make it thinner, firmer, smaller, larger, and so forth, until you can't make it any more so.

6. Let go of this sensation.

7. See if you feel a release, a balanced neutral point between the two extremes.

CHAPTER 4

Developing a Strong Mind/Body Connection

The open mind exercise you tried in the last chapter may or may not have helped change the boundaries of your ideal image. In order to make your self-image more positive, you make feeling better about yourself a habit by strengthening your mind/body connection every day. You consistently challenge yourself with new edge experiences. You can train yourself to effectively meet this challenge by systematically working with the edge in yoga poses to reconnect mind and body over and over again.

I am going to continue to use the concept of the edge to describe more thoroughly this working principle of yoga. Every teacher I have had uses the principles of the edge in some way, even though they haven't necessarily used this label for it. The edge leads you from a gross concept of a pose to a more subtle understanding, and as you refine your understanding, you strengthen your mind/body connection. Where the mind and body reconnect with each other, dead zones reawaken. When dead zones reawaken, new mind and body awareness comes to life.

To show you how this works, consider my experience in Forward Bend. As a beginner, I dreaded Forward Bend more than any other yoga pose. The mere thought of doing a Forward Bend created the sensation of a fingernail scraping a blackboard inside of my forehead. The scraping vibrated throughout the rest of my body.

Forward Bend taught me the most in yoga.

The completed pose can be done seated or standing and looks like this:

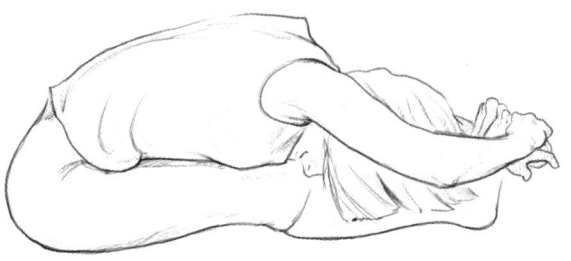

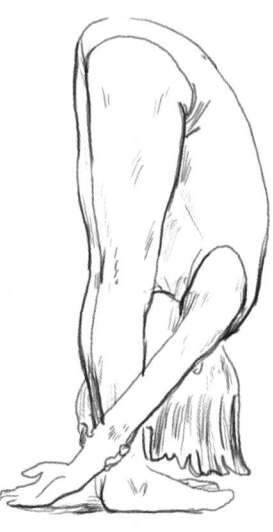

Seated Forward Bend

Standing Forward Bend

I did my first seated Forward Bends (see the first picture, above) in a class of three students at Isabelle's house. We began the pose by looping a strap around our feet and holding one end of the strap in each hand as we sat up as straight as possible (see the third picture, below). Isabelle instructed us to first focus on breathing slowly and evenly. She then guided us deeper into the pose using various points of awareness.

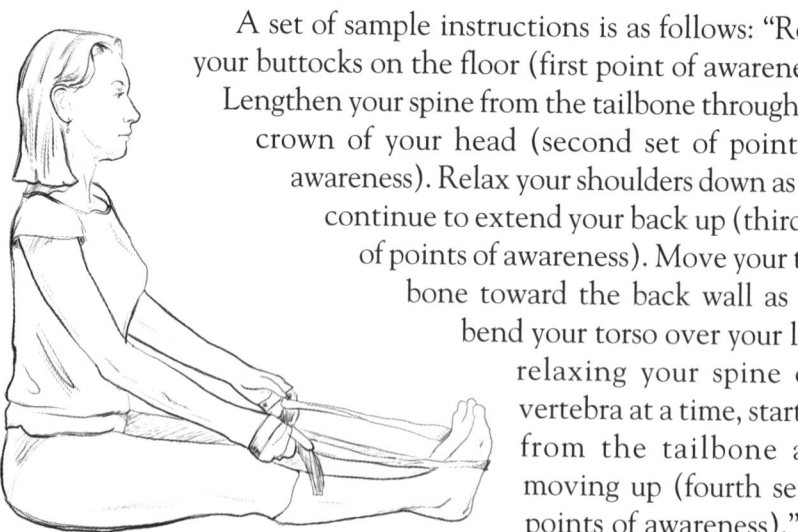

A set of sample instructions is as follows: "Relax your buttocks on the floor (first point of awareness). Lengthen your spine from the tailbone through the crown of your head (second set of points of awareness). Relax your shoulders down as you continue to extend your back up (third set of points of awareness). Move your tailbone toward the back wall as you bend your torso over your legs, relaxing your spine one vertebra at a time, starting from the tailbone and moving up (fourth set of points of awareness)."

Seated Forward Bend using a strap (for beginners)

For someone as stiff as I, who could not even get my torso verti-cal to the floor, movement forward came to an end instantly, I never even got to the part about relaxing my spine, one vertebra at a time. While my mind pictured my body lying flat against my torso in full Forward Bend, in reality I was not even sitting up straight.

I tried to bridge this gap by tugging and pulling with my arms, hunching my shoulders forward, the only parts of my body I could move, while every other part of my body tightened in response. I pulled against my own resistance. I felt like a block of concrete.

The training came in every class as Isabelle reminded us students to hold the strap with just enough pressure to bring ourselves to the edge of our ability to move without struggling. She taught us to men-tally revisit the points of awareness over and over again in the pose. And to relax and breathe deeply, lengthening our bodies in the pose on each exhalation.

As I followed her instructions and learned to stay at the edge of my tolerance, to breathe deeply and slowly, to stay focused on relax-ing my whole body, the pain I experienced in the pose subsided. I became aware of specific areas of my body that were restricting me. It was as if someone had taken a yellow marker and highlighted the areas within my body that needed my attention. These areas made their presence known in several ways, sometimes because they felt stiff and hurt or sometimes because they felt weak.

Instead of using the strap to yank myself forward using my arms and shoulders in a mindless exercise of tug-and-resist, I started to search for a sense of awareness in my tailbone, the vertebrae of my spine, my groin, the crown of my head. I searched for a mindlink to them, training them to relax and let go. When I found that link I was able to direct them to stretch out on the exhalation, slowly, without injuring myself. With this change in approach I may have only increased my outer, body extension in the pose by a minuscule amount at first, but inwardly I had taken a giant step.

My experience is a familiar one, I believe, to many yoga stu-dents. As you regularly practice a pose, bringing yourself to the edge of movement each time, breathing, relaxing within that edge, you begin to notice a transformation in your body. Over time your stiff muscles soften—like taffy that has been licked repeatedly; once rigid and inaccessible, they become soft and pliable. They become much more mobile and harbor a great deal of potential strength.

This daily focus and training of mind and body reestablishes mind/body communication. Your muscles not only gain more mobility, but they also learn to listen to your mind's direction. You reawaken dead zones in your nervous system. The mind and body learn to work as a team, as they spend time together in the pose each day, working toward a mutual goal. And because your whole body actively participates in the balance of every pose, the communication between mind and body is clear and precise.

Going back to Forward Bend, the use of excessive muscle force overcompensates for a lack of flexibility. Parts of the body (like the arms and shoulders in my example) work too hard while other parts (like the hips) are unable to move at all. Working within the edge begins to bring these body parts into balance. In a yoga pose you attend to every single part of your body; every part learns to participate in a balanced way.

This method works to increase your flexibility and strength, no matter how stiff you are. Sometimes the edge in a pose may feel as if it encompasses your whole body, which can create great reluctance to do that pose. Sometimes the thought of doing a pose can create a sensation as unpleasant as that of fingernails scraping a blackboard located somewhere in your forehead. This happens when your body is so tight that you reach the edge of many tight, inaccessible areas all at once. To counteract this sometimes overwhelming sense of reluctance you develop patience and go slowly. You learn exactly how far you can stretch into a pose without being overwhelmed. Eventually the pose you find the hardest becomes just another pose, one you can feel comfortable in, and may even enjoy.

Your struggle with body image is very much like a beginner's struggle in a difficult yoga pose. If you are not in harmony with the natural shape of your body you develop a tight, constricted view of how you should look; so there is a gap between the way you look and the image of how you want to look. Therefore, you pull and tug at yourself, you diet, exercise, buy cosmetics, wear concealing clothes, trying to get your natural shape to match your ideal image. You pull against your own natural resistance.

The practice of yoga teaches you a method for alleviating this struggle. You begin to see more possibilities. As your muscles become more flexible so does your mind; as the range of motion of your body increases, so does the range of motion of your ideas. You learn how to relax and soften an ideal image to fit around the body you have.

And you don't have to have Julie Christie's nose to do a great Forward Bend.

CHAPTER 5

Facing Anger, Fear, and Judgment

Journal Entry

Another attack of "huge stomach" today. Feeling exhausted from the constant care I need to give my mother. I am on call morning, afternoon and evening, overwhelmed by having two bodies to care for—one that is healthy and one that is sick. Sat at my desk distracted, unable to write anything worthwhile. Felt boxed in, anxious, depressed. My life, like my body, is not conforming to the image of how I think it should look. By midmorning my stomach was huge.

Stopped trying to write. I moved away from my desk, closed my eyes and concentrated on my feelings. I was angry. I let the anger build inside without trying to channel or suppress it. My jaws clenched as I pounded my stomach with my fists. "I hate you," I yelled over and over again. I thrust imaginary daggers into it, trying to deflate it. I wanted to make it small, I wanted to make it go away.

My stomach didn't go away. Strong, defiant, it stiffened in self-defense, becoming harder and rounder, warding off the blows.

Continued until I was emotionally exhausted. Anyway, it was time to pick up Neill from school.

When I returned home, I went back into my room, subdued and a little frightened by the intensity of my anger. The morning's experience shocked me into a new level of awareness. Felt cured of a certain level of self-criticism. Closed my eyes and concentrated on creating compassion for myself. I could feel a change in my posture.

I vow I will never say, "I hate my stomach" again—ever.

I promise.

I told my friend Delores about my experience, and she said, "Barbara, your stomach gets larger during the day because you have eaten." Hmm, seems I've heard that before. Still, Dolores' explanation doesn't address the essence of my experience. My stomach wasn't filled with food. It was filled with anger.

I think pent-up and repressed anger distorts the body's natural shape.

Anger is an emotion many of us are taught to deny. One time when Neill was little he had misbehaved for a whole morning, so I sent him to his room. As he stomped up the stairs, my first impulse was to discipline him for showing his anger. However, remembering a recent seminar on anger that Bob had attended, I did nothing. I let him mutter and throw things around until his ire was spent. I then went to his room and told him to fix up the mess before coming down. He did. We had a very pleasant time together for the rest of the day.

Neil's anger that day reminds me of an earlier incident when he and I were having dinner together at a restaurant. Neill had just started a new school year. As we waited for our order, he said his stomach hurt. He always complained of stomach pains during the beginning weeks of school throughout grammar school. When I asked him why his stomach hurt, he told me there were dolphins swimming around in it. The dolphins were angry. At his very young age he had a very direct awareness of the physical manifestation of his anger.

Like a lot of parents, I did not encourage him to express his anger in any way, as I was never encouraged to do so as a child. I wonder if his angry dolphins found great release, throwing things around in his room.

I think more of us should learn how to systematically and safely release anger. We spend a lot of time denying how angry we are because we don't know what to do with such strong emotions. And anger directed toward self is especially daunting and difficult to acknowledge.

The technique Bob had learned in his seminar encourages people to release the steam of anger without hurting anyone. People could have a place reserved for such releases. An "anger room" in the house, maybe, one that perhaps contains a punching bag or expendable items to throw around and smash. This way they could release the anger safely and then deal more effectively with the reasons they are angry in the first place.

The first time I deliberately vented my anger I was driving my car, late for work. My frustration was so intense I felt nauseous. When I hit the fourth red light in a row, I exploded, hurtling screams from deep inside my throat for as long as it took to exhaust myself.

When I was done, I looked out, expecting to see traffic stopped for miles, everyone staring. Instead, as I looked around I saw nothing of the sort had happened. Traffic was moving along normally, everybody going about his own business. The world had not noticed my volcanic outburst. However, my nausea vanished and I felt tremendous overall relief.

The kind of anger release I am describing is not one that encourages self-indulgence in destructive behavior. Releasing pent-up anger safely is one aspect of dealing with anger. The second aspect involves taking responsibility for the emotion and learning to detach from it.

The yoga sutras, written down by Patanjali, describe the philosophical basis of yoga practice. For nine months each year, I meet regularly with several other students to study the sutras with Debra Ann.

I, along with the other students, hit a stumbling block when several classes focused on detachment. The yoga sutras say that detachment from life's illusions—which is everything in life—decreases pain and suffering and leads to enlightenment. The problem was that detachment did not seem like a very attractive idea. How do you express love or have and achieve goals if you are detached from everything?

The book *Tuesdays with Morrie* by Mitch Albom eloquently explains the difference between detachment and indifference or sublimation of feelings. Morrie Schwartz was Mr. Albom's college professor at Brandeis University and was dying of amyotrophic lateral sclerosis, Lou Gehrig's disease. The two met every Tuesday for about three months during the last stages of Morrie's illness.

The following is an excerpt of their conversation on detachment. Morrie said,

> "Learn to detach."
>
> He opened his eyes. He exhaled. "You know what the Buddhists say? Don't cling to things, because everything is impermanent."
>
> But wait, I [Mitch] said. "Aren't you always talking about experiencing life? All the good emotions, all the bad ones?"
>
> "Yes."
>
> Well, how can you do that if you're detached?
>
> "Ah. You're thinking, Mitch. But detachment doesn't mean you don't let the experience *penetrate* you. On the contrary, you let it penetrate you *fully*. That's how you are able to leave it....You're afraid of the pain, you're afraid of the grief. You're afraid of the vulnerability that loving entails.
>
> "But by throwing yourself into these emotions, by allowing yourself to dive in, all the way, over your head even, you experience them fully and completely. You know what love is. You know what pain is. You know what grief is. And only then can you say, 'All right. I have experienced that emotion. Now I need to detach from that emotion for a moment.'"

What Morrie says about love and grief is also true for anger. At first glance the idea of letting an emotion such as anger penetrate your being may seem to have a certain element of danger to it—would you then be more likely to want to murder the idiot who cuts you off on the highway? However, I think simmering, unresolved anger probably explodes into most of the hostile encounters exemplified by road rage incidents. Safe expression of pent-up anger can be a first step to working toward resolution.

Morrie's wisdom does not encourage self-indulgence in our emotions but rather understanding and responsibility for them. We can then learn to act out of deeper wisdom and compassion.

Love and Anger Exercise

1. Sit comfortably in a chair with your feet parallel on the ground.

2. Relax and breathe naturally for five minutes.

3. Focus on your breath as it enters and leaves your body. Observe its rhythm without altering it.

4. Close your eyes and imagine yourself being someplace pleasant, or doing something you enjoy.

5. Notice how your body feels when you visualize this.

6. Shift your attention to an area of your body that you dislike. Focus on this area and notice if there is any change in your breathing, or in any other part of your body. Let your feelings come up and just stay with the breathing. Do this for a minimum of five minutes. Has your posture changed? Are you as relaxed as you were before? Are you as calm or more anxious? If your feelings get strong you can go with them for as long as you feel safe; you can also breathe deeply and release them on the exhale.

7. Take a deep breath and let go of the visualization.

8. Now focus on this same area and create a feeling of love for it. Say, "I love you." Breathe slowly and deeply. How could you show your love? Move your body into a shape to fit this feeling. Move to its rhythm; let it become a familiar dance.

Journal Entry

Fear of the dark and the abyss. I am afraid of the dark. So last night, after midnight, when everyone was asleep, I closed myself inside the laundry room. I stared into the pitch black. Waves of fear welled up in my throat. I tried to swallow them back. My throat felt like a pressure cooker about to explode. I breathed slowly and deeply to steady myself.

In the darkness, the laundry room seemed to dissolve around me, except for a small circle of the floor under my feet. Surround-

ing the circle was an abyss. I became aware of the tension in my feet. Their habitual shape stood out in bas relief. I have suction cup feet that grip onto my small circle of security. They have tightly raised arches, curled toes, and their balls and heels press firmly into the floor.

Habitual fear distorts the body's natural shape.

In a recurring dream I stand on a swaying column surrounded by the abyss. My hold on the column is tenuous, I feel that any moment I might fall off and topple into the bottomless space that lies beneath me. Eventually I wake up or go on to some other dream. However, one memorable time my dream turned, became a lucid one and I knew I was dreaming as I dreamt. I said to myself, "Barbara, you're dreaming," and stepped off the column. The column and the abyss both disappeared.

I want to live by the ocean. I can see the sun-filled room I will live in, hear the breaking of the waves, feel the weight of my dog resting against my feet as I sit at my desk, and smell the salty air through the open sliding glass doors. With such a clear image of what I want, why am I still in Colorado, looking out at the snow?

Closed my eyes to visualize this ocean scene, seeking to discover what was keeping me from it. While the visualization felt so near to me, a hair's breadth away, an abyss yawned within the gap of that tiny space.

I have read books that tell me how easy it is to create the life I want by changing my thoughts, by visualizing what I want to have. I get inspired by them for a while and then go back to my usual life. Visualizations sometimes work, sometimes they don't. Their effectiveness may depend upon whether any abysmal fears lie between you and what you want.

Michelle is a former client with a terrific wit. One day she came in excited about a self-help book she had read. "It was wonderful," she enthused, "it changed my life for a whole day." How often have you read a book, attended a seminar that really inspired you, but then never followed through with whatever exercises or other daily practices you took away from it?

Changing your life for the better can be easy with one very big qualification. You need to first confront and work through the fears that keep you from creating what you want. If you ignore this aspect you will find it very difficult to stay focused over a long enough period of time to make meaningful changes.

I don't think most of us are lazy. I think most of us are afraid.

Exercise in Fearlessness

Begin each day with a timed writing: If I weren't afraid, I would do (fill in the blank) today. Write for ten minutes. Do you have a dream that you have not done much work toward? If so, set some daily goals and use the timed writing to help you understand why you are reticent. Or you can use this timed writing with no specific goal in mind.

Journal Entry

My friend Nicki has a quirk in her ability to judge spatial relationships. After a meal, she can never judge the right-sized bowl for her leftovers. She picks a bowl that she thinks is the right size but the leftovers don't fit. I have a similar problem in my ability to judge time—it is never the right-sized receptacle for all of the "things" I want to do. I plan what I think will be a day that gets all of the routine chores on my list done with time left over for something creative or fun; instead, time always runs out before I ever finish my chores. The next day I start all over again.

One of my former electrolysis clients is a list maker. One day she came in for a treatment and announced that she was separating from her husband. She had spent the weekend cleaning out her closet, an appropriate task for that kind of life event. Tucked away in some boxes she had discovered lists she had made ten years ago. They looked almost exactly like her most recent one. She was depressed.

I am depressed, too.

I talked to Annuradha on the phone. Her son is having a hard time in school. She thinks he might have Attention Deficit Disorder (ADD). She is so tired from worrying she thinks she may have Chronic Fatigue Syndrome. I am so depressed, I am sure I have Seasonal Affective Disorder (SAD). Annuradha always runs

*out of time, too. "Maybe we have some kind of time disorder,"
she joked. Time Deficit Disorder (TDD). I like that.*

*I once visualized time as the abyss I dream about. An abyss is
a bottomless pit, something you fall through without an end. Time
is like an abyss, in a way. It has no handles to grab onto to reverse
it or slow it down. You can never take a time-out break from your
life—have it stand still for a while so you can catch your breath
until you feel more ready to continue. You can never go back in
time to redo something.*

Time is a free fall into the abyss of the unknown.

Fear changes the shape of your body. Fear that is associated with
a passing event, temporarily; chronic fear, which leads to stress and
anxiety, permanently (unless worked on and released.)

In his book *Somatics*, Thomas Hanna describes the two major
reflexes we have that protect us from danger in our environment:
one reflex is a withdrawal response, the other is a take action response. These are similar to the familiar "fight or flight" response.

He goes through a whole list of bodily responses to what he calls
the red light reflex. This is the withdrawal response to the
environment. He gives as an example a woman walking
down the street hearing a car back-
fire. Her bodily responses go from
the head down to her toes and include: the muscles of her jaw
contract, her shoulder and neck
muscles contract, her elbows bend, her
abdominal muscles contract—pulling
down her rib cage and stopping her
breathing, her knees bend, and her
ankles roll her feet inward. Her body is
flexed and crouched, ready for danger.

He then goes through a list of
bodily responses to the green light reflex. This is the take action response to
the environment. The green light reflex contracts the posterior
extensor muscles, lifting and arch-

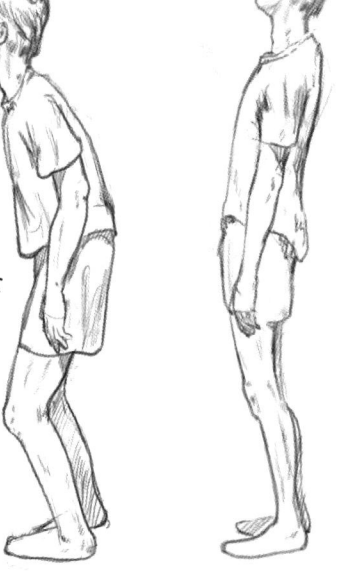

Red Light Reflex   Green Light Reflex

ing the back in a manner opposite to the crouch of the red light reflex. If the woman in the first example is confronted by a stranger who scares her and her response is to get away, some of her more specific bodily responses are that the lumbar muscles contract accompanied by a synergistic tensing of the muscles of the neck, shoulder, buttocks, and thighs.

Habitual stress leaves its imprint as a composite of these two responses. The shape of the composite depends upon how a person uniquely responds to her environment.

Posture Exercise

Observe your posture in a mirror. Stand straighter. How do you feel? Exaggerate any slouch. How do you feel?

Journal Entry

People react to you based on their life experience. Maybe even more than any innate quality you possess. No matter how hard you try; someone may not like something about you because of who they are. How they react to you is beyond your ability to control.

The yoga and qi gong have been zeroing in on the heaviness and tightness in my chest. I feel lighter, more open in my heart. I feel a new sense of vulnerability with this freedom. I would rather not judge or be judged.

A friend and I had a discussion about the difference between being judgmental toward the behavior of other people and being discerning about their behavior. We came to the conclusion that being judgmental involved our personal prejudices and biases. Being discerning was a more neutral assessment of whether or not their behavior warranted wanting to be involved with them.

"Visualize how you keep people away," Bob said. This was a technique he learned at his latest seminar. I asked him what he meant. He told me to close my eyes and do what he said. Sure enough, when I tried, I had no trouble visualizing myself surrounded by a plastic shield. I hate plastic.

I tried the visualization out on some of my friends. I was surprised, and they were too, at how easily they were able to form a picture of their emotional process. One friend, a graphic artist, pictured herself in a castle surrounded by a moat with a drawbridge that she could raise and lower at will. What a picturesque way to keep herself safe.

I think I have had my plastic shield for a long time. It insulates me from people, keeps me safe.

The journey I have undertaken to heal my self-image is a journey of my heart; I have a lot to learn about kindness and compassion. The more I practice my yoga and qi gong the more I learn to become the kind and compassionate person I want to be.

You may ask, "Don't we all need boundaries to protect ourselves?" We do. If someone were to threaten us, we would naturally want to be able to defend ourselves. Natural boundaries keep us safe but also invite people in. Natural boundaries are fluid and defined within the moment. Natural boundaries are the result of actions we take when we are in touch with our hearts and our inner wisdom.

Boundary Exercise

1. Sit in a comfortable chair with both feet resting on the ground and your hands on your knees.

2. Close your eyes and relax with deep, rhythmic breaths for about two minutes.

3. Picture how you keep other people from getting too close to you.

4. See if you can visualize how your body shape reflects how you keep people away.

Workbook Space

Describe the boundary you visualized. Is it fluid or rigid? How does it change?

CHAPTER 6

Your Body/Yourself

Journal Entry

Debra Ann's class focused on feet today. We inserted our fingers between our toes. Some of the students were flexible enough to fit their fingers between their toes as easily as a glove. I could barely get the tips of my fingers between mine, and oh, the pain in my metatarsals was sharp.

We then spread our toes wide. Curiously, my little toe and the one next to it stood together, inseparable, like two little soldiers glued together. I could not move them independently of each other.

Then we did squats, my ankles could barely move, they seemed frozen in the shape of the high heeled shoes I wore throughout my young adult life—2-inch pumps for work and 2-inch espadrilles for play. The only part of my body that looks like Barbie's—my feet.

Told my friend Len about my fear of the abyss. He said that maybe there is no abyss, that if I just keep putting one foot in front of the other, I will discover that it is an illusion. Hmmm.

Putting one foot in front of the other isn't that easy for me. I observed my tennis game today as I lost another match. I noticed the lag time between when I see the direction of the ball and when I actually move to retrieve it. Suction-cup feet are not assets on the tennis court.

When you explore the mind/body connection you discover that your body mirrors your thoughts and feelings. Your body is holographic, every part images what is happening with the whole and with every other part. This concept is the basis for such modalities as iridology and reflexology. Iridology reads the health of the body from the colors and shapes of the eye. Reflexology does so with patterns of tension in the feet or hands.

An athletic sportswear company once did an ad for sneakers explaining how the company made sneakers for everyone. The ad depicted an "athlete's foot," then two other types of foot patterns.

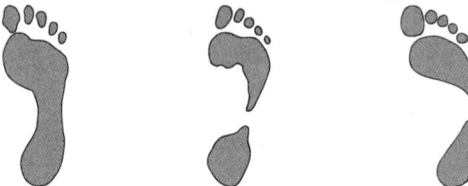

The athlete's foot looked the most relaxed and balanced touching the ground. The differences were in the arches. The other two sets of prints looked less balanced and more of the foot was not touching the ground.

The patterns below show normal, high, and flat arches.

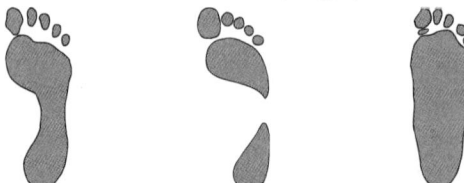

Footprint Exercises

You can observe how balanced your body is by observing the way your feet rest on the ground.

Exercise 1

You will need liquid makeup foundation and two sheets of looseleaf paper.

1. Place one of the sheets of paper on the floor near a chair.

2. Sitting on the chair, spread the foundation evenly on the bottom of one feet.

3. Stand up so that the foot with the foundation rests on the sheet of paper.

4. Close your eyes. Can you tell if you put more weight on one foot than the other?

5. Now step off the paper and see what kind of print you made. How relaxed does your footprint appear to you? What kind of arch do you have?

6. Repeat the exercise with the other foot. Does one foot touch the ground the same way as the other?

   Try this exercise a second time but first do the following: Stand on the floor with your feet hip distance apart and parallel to each other, your arms resting by your sides.

   Close your eyes and systematically relax every part of your body from your heels up to your head. Then contract your whole body as tight as you can and release.

   Repeat the exercise, noticing if there is any change in your footprints. (Do not try to manipulate your feet to even out the prints, based upon what you saw in the first set.)

   Have your footprints changed in any way?

Exercise 2

Stand as before with your feet hip distance apart, your arms by your side, and imagine how your feet would rest on the ground with great confidence and self-acceptance.

Notice and record any shifts in the rest of your body when you make the above adjustment.

Exercise 3

One winter I was struck by the contrast between two sets of footprints in the snow. I mused about the different personalities of the two people. I envisioned the first person as straightforward, focused, organized. Someone who would not be distracted once she started on a project. I envisioned the second person as a meandering person, one who might go in several directions before completing a project, one who might be more likely to go off on a tangent before they finished. What do you think?

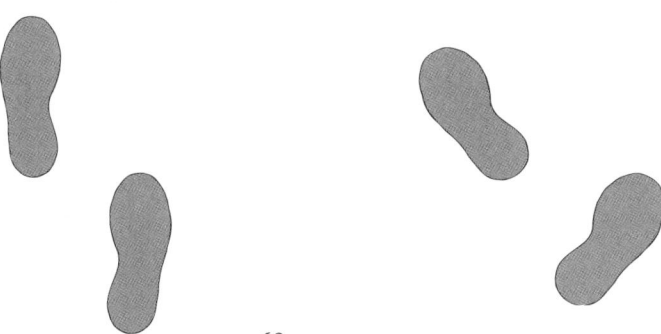

What do your footprints tell you about yourself? Try a Timed Writing exercise beginning with "My footprints say (fill in the blank)."

Journal Entry

Following the point of awareness instructions from class, I relaxed into Reclining Hero Pose. My knees felt stretched and uncomfortable. I focused on them, breathing deeply and slowly, staying within the edge of discomfort. With each exhalation, I concentrated on getting them to let go of their tension and lengthen.

Suddenly, the taste and smell of seawater invaded my nostrils as a memory played itself out. I am with my parents and my sister at the beach we visited every summer. I jump into the water and swim quickly away from the shore to impress my father, going farther out than I intend, into water that is over my head. As I stop to turn around, I realize that I can't touch bottom. I flounder in the water as my father swims to my rescue. However, the water is over my father's head, too, and as he reaches for me he loses his footing and we both go under. I feel I am drowning as seawater rushes into my nose and gaping mouth.

As I breathed slowly through the replay of this memory, a current of heat erupted from my knees and coursed through my body. The edge of discomfort softened and shifted to a new inner boundary. My knees were much more relaxed and stretched out.

The terror of this beach experience had been stored in my body, locked within my knees. It was as if my body had forgotten to let go of the terror, years after I was rescued and safe. The focus of my yoga practice unlocked and released the emotional content of the memory.

Unresolved emotional trauma distorts the body's natural shape, too.

Reclining Hero Pose

You don't have to be a daredevil to have experienced traumas that have left their marks in your body, they happen from the ordinary experiences of living—like automobile accidents, falling off slides or bicycles, tripping down stairs, pulling muscles in sports. By bringing the mind, body and emotions together to work with the distortion in the body shape that can result, yoga can help you to release old traumas and restore the resulting misalignments. When your body then releases the stagnant energy, it returns to its more natural state.

Stagnant and blocked energy from stored emotional traumas influence behavior. Yoga postures can help release stagnant and blocked energy. Many body therapies also do this. Rolfing is one such therapy.

Memory Exercise

What was a traumatic experience for you?

1. Close your eyes and breathe deeply and evenly for several minutes.

2. Revisit the experience with your mind.

3. Notice if there are any areas in your body that change when you do the above. Be especially attentive to areas of tension, anxiety, or even pain that surface.

Journal Entry

We moved quickly through a series of yoga postures in Debra Ann's class today. As we moved from one posture to the next, I noticed myself frowning, getting more upset by the minute. Everyone was out of alignment in the poses, even Debra Ann. As we continued, minute after excruciating minute, my whole body turned into one big frown.

I like to enter a pose slowly, adjusting all the minute details, so I end up as maximally aligned as possible.

Was sick with the flu earlier this week. My temperature reached 101 degrees. "I haven't been sick for quite a while," I said to Bob and Neill. "Maybe over ten years." Neill then reminded me of the year he gave me the chicken pox. Had forgotten about that— forty-two years old with the red blotches of the chicken pox all over my face on the day we were supposed to go to Dallas for our vacation.

The day before I broke out I went to work with a fever of 101 degrees. I was the salon's only electrologist; canceling my day was not an option.

My routine inner dialogue played itself out—I can't cancel my day because my schedule is full and I'm going out of town. I will disappoint everyone if I don't come in. There is nobody to help me out. I have to do it all.

Saw over twenty clients that day.

Have finally learned my lesson—I think. As dinnertime approached, got up from the love seat in our family room—told Neill and Bob they'd have to make their own dinner, reminding them of the state of my health, in case they had forgotten.

"Oh," they said in unison, startled that dinner would be their responsibility.

Went upstairs as Neill and Bob began impromptu negotiations.

Bob to Neill—You walk the dog and I'll cook.

Neill to Bob—No, I'll cook and you walk the dog.

I smiled at my son being cleverly outmaneuvered. Bob is supposed to walk the dog in the afternoon, anyway.

As I practiced Forward Bend during the next day's yoga session I felt a quantum release of tension in my lower back. A current of heat accompanied the release, coursing up from my lower back into the rest of my torso, and I was able to bend over farther than I ever had before.

Physics says that light energy is dual in nature. Sometimes it behaves like a wave vibration and sometimes like a packet of energy called a photon. It seems to me that the nature of emotional energy is similar. It can be stored in the body as a vibration which, at times, can be released in a packet of energy accompanied by a current of heat. The heat represents the freeing up of the energy that had been diverted to keep the emotion locked in.

As I broke through the resistance of allowing others to help me I felt energized. I felt that little photon of my "nobody ever helps me, I have to do it all" emotional energy pop out. I had freed up the energy it took to keep that belief and its accompanying emotions locked within my body and my life.

How did I know that letting my family make dinner was related to the release of tension in my lower back? People make connections like this all of the time.

A coworker from one of my part-time department store jobs suffered from flare-ups of tendinitis in her elbows. She didn't like the store or her job. The pain in her elbows kept getting worse until she decided to quit her job. The day after she made her decision to quit her job, the tendinitis subsided.

One of my girlfriends recognized a similar connection with chronic pain in her arm. The pain in her arm vanished after she cut down on the many hours she spent chauffeuring her two children after school. She didn't become a neglectful mother; she just brought into better balance a too-hectic routine of extra curricular activities.

I guess you could call this the psychology of the mind/body connection. Yoga is very helpful because it provides a disciplined method for making these kinds of associations. As you peel away layer after layer of the physical pain in your body, you do the same with the mental and emotional pain in your life.

Yoga poses teach you about yourself. If you are impatient with yourself in your practice, then examine how you are impatient with yourself in your life. If you don't extend yourself fully in the postures, examine where you have that tendency in your life.

Your body is the physical expression of who you are. Yoga practice helps you to become more aware of how you live your life and to develop new ways of bringing your life into balance. You then experience physical, mental, and emotional relief. Practicing yoga daily is often like having visits from your own private masseuse and therapist—all rolled up in one.

Most importantly, though, as you develop this mind/body connection you explore the inner space of your body. You learn to stay in touch with your body as the physical expression of yourself as an emotional and spiritual being. You stay more in touch with the "real you," not some object you compare to media images or societal expectations.

Mind/Body Exploration Exercise

1. Sit in a comfortable chair with both feet resting on the floor and your hands resting gently on your thighs.

2. Close your eyes.

3. What area of your life is causing you the most anxiety right now? Form a statement about what is causing this tension. Breathe for a minute and see if this is the correct statement or if a more accurate statement presents itself.

4. Scan your body from head to toe and locate the area related to this tension.

5. Focus your attention in this area for five minutes. What are your thoughts and your feelings telling you about this area? Do you see any mental images? Do you sense any smells?

6. Bring your focus back to your whole body. Open your eyes and relax for a minute or two.

7. Close your eyes a second time.

8. Think about resolving the tension in this area of your life. Make a statement about resolving this tension. Wait for a minute and see if this statement is accurate or if a more accurate one presents itself.

9. Scan your body for the area that would be most helpful in this resolution.

10. Stay focused on this area for three minutes. What are your feelings here? Do you see any mental images? Do you hear anything? What is it about this area that can help you with the tension you feel?

    Record your experience in the space provided.

Workbook Space

Journal Entry

> *Debra Ann observed my Mountain Pose today.*
>
> *She adjusted my posture, noting the bulge of my stomach. "I know," I said. "I have a lot of stuff in there."*
>
> *"You have a lot of ideas about stuff in there" she replied.*
>
> *In the evening I noticed my inner dialogue as I was making dinner. "I hope dinner comes out okay. I am sick of cooking all the time. I don't know what to make anymore. Why do I have to do it all?"*
>
> *The mind-talk descended straight to my stomach, turning it into a hard knot.*

A case can be made for the statement that our bodies are shaped by the way we experience life. For example, two of my friends are very responsible caretakers, like me. Our shoulders hurt from the brunt of that responsibility. Yet, we express our caretaker natures differently.

One of my friends is a take-charge individual. Her stance reminds me of a boxer's, somewhat hunched over, shoulders rounded forward. "Out of my way, I'll take care of everything." My other friend walks with an open chest, her shoulders pulled back: "It's okay, I'm friendly, I'll take care of you and give you what you want." My posture resembles my mother's, upper spine rounded, carrying the weight of the world on my shoulders. "I have to do it all."

People's body shapes can communicate a lot about them to the practiced eye. In the opening chapters of one book I read (I can't remember the title or author) the author described a workshop he had attended. The leader of the workshop accurately put his finger on the essence of several attendees' life experiences and relationships by observing their deportment and body shape. The leader of this workshop read a person's body like a map of that person's life.

This workshop leader had fine-tuned an ability probably all of us have. Sometimes bodily expressions of characteristics are easily recognizable. In a class I took on theme writing, the instructor assigned us the task of creating a character's face using only three physical features. Our objective was to use these features to define some aspect of the personality of the character, to make the character come to life. One student created a librarian. Her librarian had short brown hair, a wide forehead, and a no-nonsense mouth.

That last feature brought the character to life. I instantly pictured this fictitious librarian, thin lips pursed in disapproval, standing in a study room, hands on hips, impatiently tapping her foot as she admonished giggling students to be quiet.

Our bodies are the physical expression of our beings. Our bodies reflect our weaknesses and our strengths, our joys and our sorrows. When we focus on this reality we go beyond the preoccupation with our outer contours and begin to view our physical shapes with more kindly interest. We begin to see how our bodies are vehicles for self-examination and personal growth.

Mountain Pose Exercise

Mountain Pose is the basic standing posture in yoga.

1. Stand with your feet parallel to each other, hip distance apart. If you have tile or wood floors, you can line your feet up with their lines.

2. Lift your toes off the floor and spread them back down wide and long.

3. Focus on your inner heels and consciously relax them.

4. Keep your feet relaxed and spread out softly on the floor as you lift your ankles up.

5. Move your attention along the length of your legs starting at the ankles. Extend your legs from your ankles up to the top of your thighs.

6. Lift up your kneecaps to further extend and firm your thighs.

7. Relax your groin, from the center of your pubis outward.

8. Relax your tailbone. Sink it naturally toward the floor. Imagining there is a chair underneath you and you are going to sit down helps create the right movement.

9. Relax your sacrum.

10. Can you tell if your pelvic girdle tilts forward or backward? Left or right? Imagine it filled with a liquid. Would the liquid spill out the front or back and/or to one side?

11. Relax your abdomen, starting from the lower to the middle to the upper part.

12. Relax your diaphragm and rib cage, taking some deep, slow breaths.

13. Lift up your sternum; feeling the length of your spine between your sternum and tailbone.

14. Widen your shoulder blades away from the center of your spine outward.

15. Extend and lengthen your arms from the point where they meet your shoulders all the way down to the tips of your fingers.

16. Relax the palms of your hands. Relax and extend each finger toward the floor.

17. Lengthen your neck from your shoulders up through the back of your head.

18. Relax your throat

19. Relax the muscles of your jaw and then of your entire face.

20. Relax the crown of your head, feel it extend toward the ceiling. Imagine the palm of a hand on top of your head and let the crown of your head relax into it.

21. Soften your gaze.

22. Stand like this for five minutes.

23. Search your body for a place that feels comfortable and happy. Breathe slowly and deeply into that area. What does it have to say to you?

24. Search your body for a place that does not feel comfortable or happy. Breathe slowly and deeply into that area. What does it have to say to you?

25. What, if anything, do these two areas have to say to each other? Ask one first, then the other.

26. Open your eyes and look at your world with a soft gaze, as if your eyes were located at the back of your head.

Mountain Pose gives you a feel for how your body is aligned as you stand. With a straight spine and relaxed musculature, your ears, shoulders, hips and ankles all line up. Most of us stand crookedly.

Journal Entry

I could tell my shoulders have improved from the massage I got today. They have progressed from solid granite to a more porous rocklike nature. As the massage therapist kneaded the muscles I could feel little isolated granules of tension. Still, in midafternoon when I get tired, my shoulders have accumulated the most stress from the day. If I find the time to rest they release their tension like a kettle releasing steam.

One of my friends whose shoulders are still of granite quality decided she was going to release the tension in her shoulders with her mind. She wasn't very successful. It's pretty difficult to release tension you have been storing in an area for most of your life with a onetime effort of your mind. Your mind doesn't even know where to look to begin.

Storing this kind of habitual tension saps the energy from your body. Curl your fingers into a tight fist. Now imagine walking around all day keeping that fist tight. In a way, that is what you are doing with habitually tight muscles in your body. You are expending that kind of energy.

Downward-Facing Dog Exercise

Downward-Facing Dog is a great pose for the shoulders.

1. Make sure you are on a non-skid surface such as a hardwood or linoleum floor or a yoga mat.

2. Kneel on your hands and knees, placing your hands slightly forward from your shoulders and a little wider than shoulder width apart.

3. Adjust your knees so that they are the width of and directly under your hips. Curl your toes (see position1).

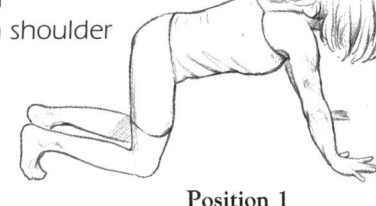

Position 1

4. Spread your fingers wide and adjust them so that the middle finger of each hand faces directly forward.

5. Inhale and on the exhale relax your neck and shoulders.

6. Sink your palms into the floor and raise your wrists away from your hands.

7. Breathe deeply and evenly as you elongate from your wrists up through your lower arms, through your elbows, through your upper arms and through your shoulders.

8. Relax and elongate along your back up through your hips, bringing your buttocks back toward your heels (see position 2)

Position 2

9. Inhale and on the exhale lift your hips up by moving your thighs and buttocks away from your head, straightening your legs. Bring your heels down to the floor as you firm your knees (see position 3).

10. Breathe deeply and evenly for ten slow breaths. As you do, continue to move your thighs and buttocks away from your head. You want your legs, not your shoulders, to bear the weight of your body.

Position 3

11. If you feel you have stayed in the pose long enough, come down into Child's Pose—step 15. To stretch more deeply, inhale and on the exhale bend your knees and bring your torso toward your legs.

12. Keep your torso in place and on your next exhale straighten your legs and bring your heels back down to the floor.

13. Breathe evenly and deeply for another five breaths.

14. Repeat steps 11 through 13 one more time and then go directly to step 15.

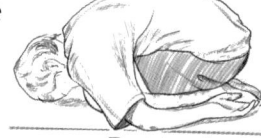

Position 4

15. Bring your knees to the floor, spread them wider, and curl into Child's Pose (see position 4).

CHAPTER 7

Development of Inner Poise—The Secret to a New Self-Image

Molly was a college friend. I remember her as very tall and thin, with feet and hands that looked somewhat large and gangly—my judgment, I know. Molly went through a startling transformation toward the end of our senior year. Ready to graduate from four successful years of college, engaged to our tall, thin, handsome astronomy teacher (a graduate student), and with a great job opportunity ahead of her, her life took on a rosy hue.

One day close to graduation, as she was describing the logistics of her life, I stared at Molly in surprise. She was beautiful. Her blonde hair shimmered, her complexion was radiant, and her feet and hands somehow no longer looked large and awkward. She glowed with a rosy hue. Molly's transformation was so startling that to this day I remember how she looked more than I remember anything we said or did together.

Delores remembers a period in her life when she experienced the same kind of inner peace and glowed like Molly did. So do I. We were happy because our lives were so wonderful at the time because we had what we desired. It was easy to be content and focused in the present. It was easy to eat healthy foods and keep physically fit. Of course, as time moved on and things changed, our equilibrium and peace, our happiness in the present moment vanished, vanquished by the changing circumstances in our lives.

This is not to say Delores and I never experienced peace and tranquility again; however, the special time for us, when life was so rosy, gave us a taste of what true inner poise is like. When you develop the wisdom that comes from inner poise your life does become a little like a rose garden. You are able to meet your challenges, enjoy, and develop your gifts more easily.

Inner poise develops wisdom. Wisdom brings self-acceptance and equanimity. With the development of self-acceptance and equanimity your life takes on a new shape around you. Inner poise develops inner peace. Think of how differently your day goes if you have had a good night's sleep or a restless sleep. The difference between inner peace and the lack of it, is akin to this contrast. You respond to life's events less from fear, anger, and judgment and more from confidence, compassion, and knowledge. Your decisions become more adventurous and courageous.

You develop inner poise when you become fully attentive to what is happening now. Your life is happening now. Your body is a dynamic process, continually changing from one moment to the next. If nothing else, it is one moment older. But its weight and shape vary from day to day, depending upon your menstrual cycle, the season, and many other factors. An ideal body shape is an illusion. Illusions disappear when you are living your life focused in the present.

You become more poised with the strong mind/body connection you develop through yoga practice. As your body and mind work together in yoga, focused on what you are experiencing in the moment in a pose, your inner sense of well-being and self-acceptance grows stronger. As your sense of well-being and self-acceptance grows stronger, media images and current beauty fads will have a less harmful effect on you.

Inner poise is not magically bestowed upon you when media images change or beauty fads are eliminated. You cultivate it with discipline and focused intent. Discipline and focused intent require you to work toward your goal daily. You replace an old habit of anxious response to media images or other outside cues for self-acceptance with a new habit of restful self-awareness that comes from a centered wisdom within you.

In order to replace an old habit with a new one, you must really desire to change and have an ongoing commitment to it. You need to be vigilant and diligent. Yoga discipline is a tool that reminds you daily of your goal. It helps you to follow through with your commitment.

Journal Entry

We did Cobbler's Pose with our backs aligned against the wall in class. Debra Ann went around the studio adjusting our postures. When she came to me, she pressed her hands on my outer hipbones. "Bring your mind here, into your hips," she commanded. I was perplexed. Concentrating as hard as I was, my mind, whatever there was of it, should already be in my hips. I focused on the pressure of her hands on my hipbones.

Suddenly I felt a higher level of awareness in my hips. My mind dropped down from my head and landed in my hips with what sounded to me like an audible "ka thunk." "That's it!" Debra Ann exclaimed, knowing my mind had found its way into my hips as surely as you would know someone was home if you saw them there through their window. Satisfied, she moved on to the next student.

What is it like for your mind to be present where it wasn't before? To use a Yogi Berra–esque witticism, "You ain't there until you've been there." Experiencing a heightened level of awareness in a body part changes your perception of it. The difference is like thinking about visiting France, reading books about France, calling a travel agent to find out about fares to France, and actually getting on a plane and visiting the country. This heightened awareness has the same sense of discovery as finding that less-traveled meandering neighborhood street.

Over and over again I visit a part of my body that had been closed off to conscious awareness and my surprise is that I wasn't aware of the blockage until I could visit the area with awareness and feel the difference.

How did Debra Ann know my mind wasn't in my hips just by looking at them? She must have X-ray vision. She knows where your mind is present and where it isn't present. She can see where your energy flow is blocked. She sees the interrelationship of all of the parts of the body; when one part of the body is out of alignment, other parts adjust to compensate and also become unaligned. Sometimes she instructs you to adjust one part of your body in order to effect the release of another. Her gift seems magical at times.

So much of yoga practice is like this experience. Until you reach a new depth of awareness, you have nothing to compare against. In classes teachers will repeat essentially the same elements of a pose over and over again. You just keep following the instructions to the extent of your ability and over time what you are actually doing in a pose changes dramatically.

We often spend our time and focus in some parts of our body, neglecting others. I spend a lot of time thinking. I am most familiar with the world from my head's perspective. When I tried this next exercise and shifted the focus of my awareness into my heart, I noticed a profound change. My stream of disjointed thoughts, filled with worries and anxieties, vanished instantly. My heart's view of the world was calm and silent.

Body Awareness Exercises

Exercise 1

1. Sit comfortably in a chair with your feet resting on the floor and parallel to each other. Rest your hands lightly on your thighs.

2. Close your eyes and focus on your breath. Do not change its rhythm. Just be aware of it.

3. Say, "I am exhaling" on the exhalation and "I am inhaling "on the inhalation. Do this for three minutes.

4. Next, focus your attention on your heart. Continue breathing evenly and see if you notice any change in how you feel when you do this. Can you tell what your heart area is like? Does it feel open or closed? Is it tight or relaxed? Are you comfortable there or not?

5. Open your eyes, still focusing on your heart. As you look out at the world from your heart, is your perception of it any different? Do you frequently or infrequently view the world from your heart?

6. Try doing this exercise focusing on other areas of your body. Bring your focus to your gut, your stomach, or your reproductive area. Record your experiences in the space provided.

Exercise 2

Where in your body do you spend most of your time? Stop at various times during the day to discover where your focus is. Shift your awareness to different areas of your body. Notice any changes in your mood, outlook, or physical well-being when you do this. Especially see if you can make a shift when you are feeling stressed—angry, anxious, fearful, and so forth—locate an area in your body that feels differently and focus on that area. See if doing this exercise helps you change the feeling.

The next exercise is helpful to get a feel for how much conscious awareness you have in your feet and hands.

Exercise 3

You need your feet bare for this one.

1. Sit on a carpeted floor or mat.

2. Insert the fingers of your right hand in between the toes of your left foot for as far as your fingers can go.

3. Squeeze your toes with all five fingers.

4. Squeeze your fingers with all five toes.

   Are you able to squeeze all of your toes and all of your fingers or do some of them not respond to your conscious instructions?

   Notice how precise and clear you can communicate with your fingers and toes. Take note if you in any way tense or activate other parts of your body in addition to or instead of your toes and fingers.

5. Try the same exercise with your left hand and right foot.

Record your experience on the page provided.

Workbook Space

Journal Entry

I don't use the muscles of my lower back in headstand. My abdominal and shoulder muscles compensate. They try to do all the work. They contract tightly to hold me up as my lower back sags and my tailbone sticks out. This is how I stand right side up. My abdomen has to struggle against gravity to keep me from falling over (it has to do it all, while my lower back is out to lunch). Being upside down in headstand shows me how I stand right side up.

Yoga poses teach you to observe not only your physical but also your mental and emotional habits. As you learn to observe yourself in yoga, you learn to observe yourself in daily life.

Like the time our friend Danny needed to visit a hospital in Denver and stayed with us for four days. He brought a friend who was a talking head. This friend of our friend knew everything about everything. He really did. The whole family found him exhausting. Midway through the visit, we were looking forward to him leaving.

I went to yoga class and then to a coffee shop. As I drank my coffee and contemplated our visitor I realized how tightly I was holding onto the expectation that everybody should behave in a way that made me comfortable. I was not leaving room for all of us to just be, vibrant human beings responding to the energy patterns created by being together, doing the best we can.

I observed the expectation I was holding onto and the anxiety it created from the calm perspective carried over from class. The expectation felt like a mental crust formed from a stiff part of my brain. The brain has dead zones, too.

As I made this somewhat detached observation of myself, the mental crust dissolved and my attitude softened. My anxiety around the visit receded.

The experience was similar to the work done in a yoga pose, stretching the muscles in my hamstrings or upper back and relaxing them to release their tension. This time, instead of physical stiffness, I stretched and relaxed my stiff approach. I expanded my mental range of motion.

Yoga is as good for the brain as it is for the muscles of the body; it reveals the tightness of your thoughts and shows you where you need to be more flexible. Yogis say you should strive for equanimity. Michael Lee likened life's situations to yoga poses. "Hold the pose, you'll figure it out," he once quipped.

You develop the ability to observe yourself when you follow the points of awareness that lead you into a pose. You follow your teacher's instructions to the best of your ability. For example, in Triangle Pose (you can try the pose at the end of this section) a sample set of instructions are as follows.

1. Stand with your feet about 3 to 3½ feet apart and parallel to each other.

2. Raise and extend your arms at shoulder height

3. Turn your right foot out at a 90-degree angle to your right, and your left foot slightly in.

4. Make sure your big toes are relaxed and stretched out completely on the floor (big toes have a habit of popping up in Triangle Pose).

5. Firm your thighs, pulling your kneecaps up to maintain the strength in your legs throughout the pose.

6. Straighten any tilt in your pelvis by relaxing your sacrum and letting your tailbone rest naturally toward the floor.

7. Exhale and extend your torso over your right leg and place the palm of your hand on the floor or any part of your leg that it reaches.

8. Extend your left arm toward the ceiling.

9. Extend your arms by imagining two people pulling your fingers from opposite directions.

10. Look up at your left thumb.

These are just a sampling of the instructions, or points of awareness, that guide you into the pose.

As you maintain the pose for a while, your body tends to shift. When you bring your focus back to the points of awareness you started with, your body parts are no longer aligned in the manner in which you originally arranged them. Your big toe may be sticking up instead of stretched out on the floor, or your pelvis may be tilted so that your tailbone sticks out, or you may have lost the strength in your legs.

So you start all over again, readjusting your toes, your pelvis, your legs. These points of awareness are the building blocks of the mind/body connection.

When your mind/body connection is weak, you feel like a juggler in a pose. You get your big toe to rest on the floor and then turn your attention to adjust the tilt in your pelvis, then check out your kneecaps. When you have completed your round of adjustments and return to the beginning you find your body parts distracted, no longer aligned as you had left them. They have forgotten what they should be doing. They are (metaphorically) staring off into space, or involved in some other activity instead of performing their roles. You have to patiently reposition them.

As you continue this process day in and day out, a wonderful transformation takes place. Your body gains in strength and flexibility and awareness. Your range of motion increases and your body parts are more comfortable in their roles. When you adjust one body part, a certain level of awareness remains, even when the main focus of your attention is elsewhere. Your big toe continues to rest, relaxed on the floor, your pelvis remains straight, and your kneecaps keep their adjustment—your legs strong for the duration of the pose.

These parts of your body are now like actors who have become proficient in their roles. Your conscious awareness has expanded and your mind/body connection has become much stronger. The connection becomes so strong, that your body's memory of being strong and aligned during your yoga practice carries over into your everyday life. As you go about your daily routines your body is filled with awareness and stays strong, relaxed, connected, just as you trained it to be in a yoga pose. Your natural intelligence shines through in all of your everyday activities.

This process builds the foundation of inner poise.

Triangle Pose Exercise

1. Stand with your feet about 3 to 3½ feet apart, parallel to each other, toes facing forward (see position 1).

2. Lift up the front of your right foot, spread your metatarsals wide and then reposition your foot back on the floor, elongating your toes.

3. Lift up the back of your right foot, relax and spread your heel wide, repositioning it back on the floor.

4. Do steps 2 and 3 with your left foot.

5. Extend your arms out at shoulder height.

Position 1

6. Rotate your right foot out at a 90-degree angle.

7. Rotate your left foot in at about a 30 degree angle (see position 2).

8. Lift up your kneecaps and firm your thighs.

9. Relax your shoulders down toward the floor.

10. Relax your sacrum and extend your tailbone toward the floor.

11. Lengthen and extend your torso over your right leg and bring your right hand to rest on the floor or whatever part of your right leg you can reach.

12. Look up at your left hand with your right eye (see position 3).

Position 2

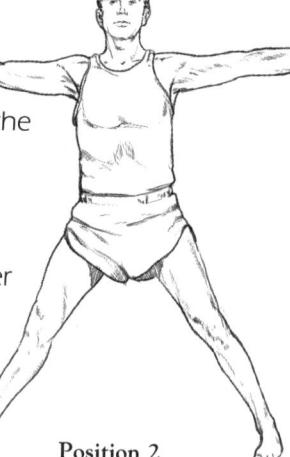

13. Inhale and exhale deeply for several moments.

14. Bring your focus back to your left foot and notice if it has shifted, especially note if its outer edge is still completely resting on the floor.

15. Bring your attention to your right foot. Notice if your big toe is still resting completely on the floor.

16. Bring your focus back to your pelvis. Has its position shifted? If so, readjust it so that it is in a neutral position, neither tilting forward nor backward.

17. Do your legs feel strong in the pose?

18. Inhale and come up, returning to position 2.

19. Bring your feet parallel to each other again.

20. Repeat the pose to the opposite side. Begin with step 6 and end with step 19.

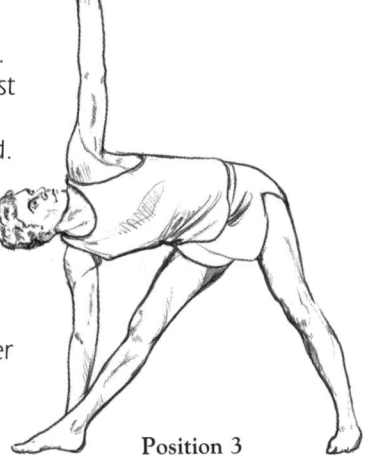

Position 3

21. Bring your feet together and stand quietly in Mountain Pose for a moment.

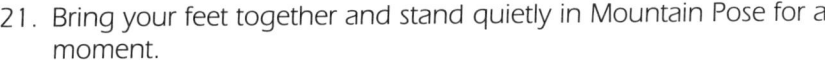

CHAPTER 8

Inner Poise
and Courage

The biggest obstacle you will probably encounter in changing your self-image is your fear. Fear of change, fear of the unknown, fear that the life you create with a different self-image might be worse than what you have now. Navigating through the wilderness of transformation takes courage.

People have courage in different areas of their lives. You may be courageous in areas that I am not and I may be courageous in areas that you are not. When we are self-confident we have the most courage; we trust our ability to handle a variety of outcomes to a situation. When we are insecure, we have less courage; we are more likely to latch upon only one outcome as safe or acceptable.

The discipline of yoga builds self-confidence and teaches equanimity. Equanimity is the ability to stay focused in the present and accept whatever outcome comes from your decisions and actions. You become more courageous this way.

Remember: The wisdom of the ages tells us to let go. It is our fears that whisper we cannot and create a thousand different reasons why we shouldn't.

Journal Entry

> *Told my family I was sick and tired of doing everything and that they were going to have to help out more. Neill decided he would wash his own clothes. The first few times he started up the stairs with his laundry basket I felt guilt—and something else I didn't immediately identify. He looked so mature with that basket of laundry that I changed my mind, telling him I'd do it for him. But he wouldn't let me.*
>
> *The something else—relinquishing the chore of doing my son's laundry—brought up anxiety that I hadn't expected. It felt as if the status of our whole relationship was at stake. I was face-to-face with my diminishing role as the mother of a dependent child.*
>
> *For a couple of days our cat changed his daily behavior. He spent one afternoon sleeping under my father's bed; he spent the next afternoon outside, not coming into the house as he usually does, to nibble on his dry cat food, or get a drink of water, or stretch out on his favorite pillow. I was perturbed. Was he sick? Maybe he didn't like us anymore and would look for another home.*

The observation that we want our lives to be different, but we don't want to change, has a corollary: We may want our world to change around us, but only in the narrow, prescribed manner we have in mind. That's why we may be more ambivalent to the changes we think we want than we consciously recognize. We may want some but not all of the changes that a transformation embodies. We are reluctant to face the unpredictable effects a new sense of self and its attendant new behaviors will bring.

When you change your self-image, you are different; you change other people's perceptions and responses to you. This process can be disconcerting because you have no control over how they will react to the "new" you.

Relationships can be like a tennis match. The tennis ball bounces back and forth from one court to the other. You may hit a smashing return over the net thinking you've finally figured it all out, but instead the ball comes back at you harder and faster.

Often it does seem easier to just sit back and complain instead.

Journal Entry

I had defrosted some fish and was opening a jar of brown rice for dinner last Wednesday. Bob suggested we go out to eat. I started to object—oh no, that's okay, I'm already making dinner—when I stopped myself. Where is that part of me that said that? I quickly put away the rice and fish and we went out.

Why is change so hard? I think of the Phoenix, symbol of transformation, crashing and burning, then rising up from the ashes. More often, though, you struggle to change your life over time. Transformation is drawn out and smelly, like the garbage rotting in a compost heap. When you come through it though, your life becomes sweeter and fresher, like the fresh-smelling humus that nourishes new growth.

I worked at the same department store during Christmas this year. I ended up in women's lingerie. One day I was planted at the cash register in the middle of the floor and faced a nonstop stream of shoppers for my entire eight-hour shift. After a while I felt like a duck sitting as a target in a firing range.

When the holidays were over I vowed I would never work there again. "Oh, Barbara, you've said that before." Nicki dismissed me with a laugh. I was hurt and a little annoyed. Then Lynn laughed, too, when I told her. Hmmm, I don't remember telling them I definitely would never work there again, ever. Even if I did, I was probably just griping.

This time I really mean it—I will never go back (barring I don't need a job to fend off destitution.)

I have wondered where intent comes from. I observe that my friends and myself often struggle repeatedly with the same challenges. We resolve that things will be different, and they are for a while, but then we end up pretty close to where we were before. If we all have free will, then why do we spend so much time doing things we don't want to do?

Yoga texts teach that we all have the seed of enlightenment within. In his book The Five Stages of the Soul, Dr. Moody says all traditions teach we have an essence, a core within us that we have forgotten about. This core is covered up by the distractions of the material world.

If there is an instinct, an inner desire to express our natural selves, to create harmonious lives, then maybe intent comes when that desire is strong enough.

Debra Ann's take on the matter was very practical. She said that we do things that bring us unwanted results over and over again until we get tired enough of it to stop.

In her book *The Dance of Anger*, Harriet Lerner identifies what she calls the "change back" reaction. When one family member significantly changes her role in the family dance, other members will try to make her change back so that they will all feel secure. I think we also at times have our own internal change-back mechanism.

Life changes can be tricky. True change comes from inside, not necessarily from how you change your environment. One of my clients was the co-owner of a very successful business. She sold out her partnership because she had no time for herself. Three months later she was helping her boyfriend start a new hotel business in Montana (she lived in Denver). Every Friday she drove for ten hours to spend the weekend there to help out. Again she had no time for herself. She was a little closer to creating what she wanted but I think she was still struggling with her own change-back reaction. Sometimes we're not really totally sure we want to go through with the changes we think we want because we know we will be upsetting the apple cart for a while.

Change takes time and happens in increments. Another client of mine was married to a husband who physically abused her. She divorced him and then married someone who verbally abused her. When I first met her she had divorced her second husband and was involved with the most wonderful and attentive man in the world. Three months later, after they began dating exclusively, he was ignoring her because he was so involved in his business. I didn't see her after that but I hope she eventually got what she wanted; she seemed to be zeroing in on it.

Autobiography In Five Short Chapters
by Portia Nelson

CHAPTER ONE
I walk down the street.
> There is a deep hole in the sidewalk.
> I fall in.
> I am lost...I am helpless.
>> It isn't my fault.
It takes forever to find a way out.

CHAPTER TWO
I walk down the street.
> There is a deep hole in the sidewalk.
> I pretend I don't see it.
> I fall in again.
> I can't believe I am in the same place.
>> But, it isn't my fault.
It still takes a long time to get out.

CHAPTER THREE
I walk down the same street.
> There is a deep hole in the sidewalk.
> I see it is there.
> I still fall in...it's a habit...but,
>> my eyes are open.
>> I know where I am.
It is *my* fault.
I get out immediately.

CHAPTER FOUR
I walk down the same street.
> There is a deep hole in the sidewalk.
> I walk around it.

CHAPTER FIVE
I walk down another street.

Journal Entry

I stopped practicing for a week when we went to Mexico. I was disappointed at how much ground I had lost in Forward Bend in that short time. I felt like a beginner again, even though I really did not revert back to anywhere near how tight I originally was in the pose. Still, my habitual way of handling life, reflected in my body, hasn't changed as much as I would have liked it to.

I had a glass and a half of wine at lunch with Lynn. When we were in the restaurant parking lot I demonstrated my Forward Bend, proud that I could almost put my palms on the ground. I not only put my palms on the ground, I did so easily with elbows bent. There is nothing like a glass of wine for instant equanimity and relaxation. It showed me that even though I have stretched out and lengthened my body, I have not completely incorporated this new habit of length into my daily life.

I don't think you can discount how much your body reflects how you have chosen to lead your life. I remember scraping my back raw as a child. When visiting my maternal grandparents I would often go next door to visit their neighbor's daughter, who was a year older than I was. One day when my friend wasn't home I received permission to use her swing, a homemade one attached to a tree. I swung higher and higher, feeling joyful and free—until I fell off. My left foot became entangled in the swing, dragging me along as my back scraped along the gravel underneath.

When I concentrate, the memory of that trauma feels bristly, like a hairshirt on my back. Like other habitual physical discomforts, I am not aware of the sensation as I carry on with my daily activities. But when I sit quietly and focus I am aware of the bristly feeling on the surface of my skin.

I came away from the experience feeling that swinging high is dangerous and dumb. I didn't want to try that again for a long time. I developed an extremely cautious approach to life as well. I mentally took that adventurous but dumb little girl and imprisoned her for her own good. I think my stiff ankles and tight back reflect this choice.

I have gotten better at experimenting with my adventurous nature; however as I work my way through the physical and emotional traumas I have experienced, remnants still remain.

CHAPTER 9

The Usual
Suspects

The biggest weapon you have for counteracting your fears is to acknowledge them and take responsibility for making changes in your life. Friends debate with me about who we should blame for our body image problems. I know I am as guilty as the next person of not wanting to take responsibility. However, I do think that improving our body images is up to us, even if outside forces beyond our control often appear to be "doing it to us."

Here are some real-life quotes, with the names changed to protect the innocent—and my friendships.

Chris: "A man tells you he loves you and then you see the way he looks at an attractive woman and you don't believe in yourself anymore."

Megan: "We are products of society. Look at how differently people look and behave in different cultures."

Kim: "We think we should look a certain way because of the pictures we see in magazines and on television."

Denise: "The pictures of thin glamorous models make us feel insecure."

Lisa: "Of course it's their fault."

Round up the usual suspects.

It has been pointed out that a rounder, fuller female body was considered beautiful during the painter Rubens' time. Imagine how unfortunate all the skinny, flat-stomached women were then.

Having a list of suspects has its benefits. You can gripe to your friends about the media, society, and men, and feel comforted that if only they would change, things would be better. Commiserating over a list of suspects feels really good. However, for meaningful long-term body image changes we need to examine ourselves, because each of us has a unique path to self-acceptance.

The reason I listed the quotes is that you can see how the outlooks vary. I think the differences in perspective show different kinds of self-doubts, even if in general we are mostly vulnerable because we want to be accepted, respected, and found attractive.

Our fears and vulnerability to criticism affect how we respond to others. By getting to the basics, by acknowledging our fears and vulnerability, we lay the groundwork for developing more positive body images. Body image reflects self-image. Most of us know people who are attractive even though they are not conventionally beautiful. This type of beauty is the "inner beauty" all of us want. Most of us listen to what society wants us to do in some areas of our lives but not others. In areas where we are confident, we are comfortable, even proud to be different and unique.

In like manner, most of us have some if not many parts of our bodies that do not match the conventional standard of beauty and yet we don't obsess about them all.

Journal Entry

Monday morning. Had an argument with Bob. Went into my room and sulked. Debated whether or not to resort to the "I" rule for some resolution. The "I" rule would illuminate my role in the fight and lead to understanding and reconciliation. Sick and tired of the "I" rule.

Please God, just for once, let it be completely Bob's fault.

Bob learned about the "I" rule at the last seminar he attended. It states that when you are evaluating your role in an interaction you have to start your sentences with the word "I." The rule is meant to help you to take responsibility for your part in your marital (or other relationship) conflicts. A sentence such as "I have to do all the work in the house because I married someone who doesn't help out," even though it contains two "I's" is incorrect. You are not supposed to ignore your responsibility and blame someone else.

Bob and I seem to argue over the same themes time after time. We are not alone. I read that a lot of married couples repeatedly argue over the same issues. The familiar pattern of angry interaction often takes you by surprise; it happens any time, anywhere. As my friend Delores observed, you could be watching TV, discussing the weather, when your conversation evolves into your relationship. Harriet Lerner calls this phenomenon "the dance of anger" in her book by that name. She says relationships are a dance. People dance together in the same pattern over and over again, and each one contributes.

When there is conflict the relationship becomes an angry dance. You can change your relationship's dance of anger by acknowledging your own role in it. If your partner changes with you, you continue to dance together. If he doesn't want to change, you may have to step on his toes until he does, or your relationship may come to a natural end. A death, of sorts. Your dance partner may be a spouse, but it can be anyone or anything in your life—your lover, a coworker, your child, your job, society, or the media.

Monday evening. Got past feeling sorry for myself and acknowledged the more subtle feelings that contributed to my part in the argument. Felt much better. Bob later owned up to his share of the blame. When Bob and I both take responsibility for our contribution to a conflict our marriage works better.

I have (mostly) given up trying to change my husband. Trying to change anyone or anything—men, society, the media, or even other women I know—is like Brer Rabbit trying to teach the tar baby manners. The more Brer Rabbit hit that tar baby, the more deeply he became embedded in its black morass.

When you assume more responsibility for your role in a relationship, your "I" sentences become more insightful. For example, a sentence such as "I do all the work in the house because I married someone who doesn't help out," becomes "I do all the work in the house because I am afraid if I don't, everyone will desert me." The more you own your feelings, the less angry you are toward anyone else and the more you understand yourself.

If you want to be happy with yourself and your body you need to go below surface appearance and investigate your more subtle feelings and motivations. When you look inside yourself for answers, you grow in wisdom; you react differently to the people and events in your life. As your perspective deepens, the people and situations that once made you angry or self-conscious or insecure no longer do. Your growth in perspective changes them in a way that has nothing to do with making them different. You transform them from people and events that once evoked self-consciousness or insecurity to people or events that do not. Like magic.

The magic formula for transforming relationships is: *change of self equals change in personal relationships.*

This is an unfailing formula for all relationships, including collective ones like society or the media, and so forth. Your family, friends, and coworkers may make changes in their lives based upon your new attitude, but only if they are willing. If your objective depends upon transformation of others, then your success depends upon them. With this formula, your success is up to you.

It sure beats the tar baby.

Whether or not you learn to love and accept your body does not involve the transformation of any person except you. When you tire of fantasizing about an image you cannot live up to, you alone have the power to make the change. You do not waste energy trying to manipulate anyone or anything around you but instead focus on your own personal growth. This responsibility is probably enough to give anyone all of the challenge she can handle.

> "I thought I could change the world. It took me a hundred years to figure out I *can't* change the world. I can only change Bessie. And, honey, that ain't easy, either."—quote from Bessie Delany, 101 years old when the book *Having Our Say: The Delany Sisters' First 100 Years* was written.

The Power of "I" Exercise

When an opportunity arises, make up your own "I" sentences, remembering that they need to be statements about you, how you are feeling, and what you are thinking.

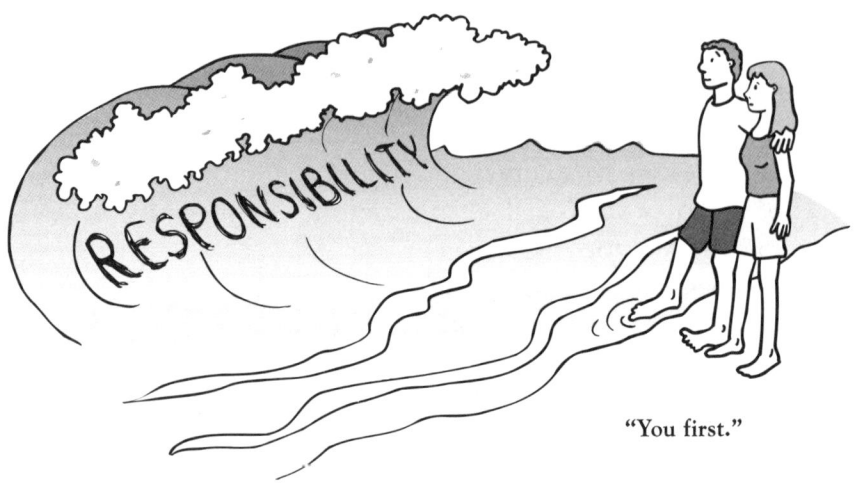

"You first."

Journal Entry

Yesterday Bob was late getting home. My thoughts wandered to what life would be like without him. I was engulfed by overwhelming sadness and loneliness. Neill goes to college next year. I pictured myself alone, an eccentric old lady living with my father, dog, and cat. The emotions were as real as if these events had already happened.

I think that the feelings of loneliness and abandonment are already inside of me, even though I have not been abandoned. How else could I know and feel them in such depth? A friend of mine, a successful businesswoman, sees herself as a bag lady. To her, a bag lady means being alone, unable to take care of herself, having no social stature. Friends have told her how unlikely she is ever to be a bag lady. Yet, in spite of her success, she is a bag lady inside.

If people tell you how intelligent, how attractive, how artistic you are but you don't believe them, if instead you dwell on the one person, whoever it is, who tells you the opposite, then that mes-

sage activates an emotionally charged thought that is already within you. That message is the one you really believe. Likewise, if people around you say you cannot succeed at something and yet you persist because you believe you can, then no matter how loud their message is you don't listen because your belief in yourself is what resonates within you.

My friend Nicki and I have spent hours debating whether our cultural views of what makes the body beautiful engender self-doubt and a negative body image in young girls, who otherwise would be perfectly okay with themselves. Think about the relationship a baby has with her body. She does not know she is separate from it. She is closer to her natural state of harmony with her body. She has no image to live up to—yet. So, how did the image get there?

I believe nothing is ever 100 percent one way all of the time, still I don't understand how, an "I'm okay" feeling becomes an "I'm not okay" feeling if a person didn't have some self-doubt to begin with. I emotionally resist the notion that there may have been no initial self-doubt. I don't like to think I may have had something "put into me" that wasn't already there. To engender self-doubt that wasn't there already in some form seems to negate free will and self-determination. And anyway, who among us doesn't have some kernel of self-doubt?

However the case may be, my friend and I agree that we can choose to change how we respond to the input we get. Societal images of the body beautiful will probably always be plentiful. I'm not sure it is even practical to campaign for more realistic media images per se. Clothes manufacturers, cosmetics companies, and all the other vendors who advertise want to sell their products and it is in their self-interest to create attractive pictures. Any beautiful picture in a magazine, any beautiful model on TV would resemble the body type of some people and leave others out.

Therefore, my advice is to make your view of your body your responsibility. The people you encounter and the society you live in play a tune with what is within, however it happened to get there. Taking responsibility for your feelings gives you the greatest power in the world—the power to change yourself. I believe this is the most effective way of changing the world around you.

Journal Entry

This past month I have focused on the hardest elements of my yoga practice, those that make me feel the most weak or afraid. Not surprisingly, I have also focused on doing whatever else in my life makes me feel weak or afraid.

For the first time I have been able to relax in Forward Bend. Up until now the pose has been a form I had to conquer by rigidly lining up all of its elements and enduring. Forward Bend has been the hardest pose for the longest time because of the tightness in the back of my body—from the back of my scalp down to the backs of my heels. Sometimes I picture my back to be like a congealed engine block.

Bob finished reading a book that describes how successful people often create imaginary councils of advisors for help in making their decisions and creating wealth. These advisors take on a life of their own, like the characters in a novel often do. A council of advisors seemed like a great idea. I decided to create an imaginary council, too.

I created an advisor to help me organize my work, an advisor to help me make money, and an advisor to oversee how I would invest all of the money I would make. As I started to call my council to order, a caged young girl, locked up somewhere within my abdomen, interrupted my proceedings.

"I want you to buy me a swing," she said.

"Go away, don't bother me," I scolded her, "Can't you see I'm busy organizing my new life?"

"You won't have a new life, if you don't pay attention to me," she replied.

I vividly remember a lunch date with Kathy, a client I hadn't seen in several years. When I knew her as a client she was in a long-term unsatisfying relationship. When we met she had ended it. She had reconnected and was living with someone she had been in love with in high school. She said that for a long time she had imagined herself with someone new, happy with life. But that person who dreamed of a more fulfilling relationship then was not the person she was now. She had to go through a transformation first. Her "old self" could not have created her new life.

It took me four agonizing years to get up enough courage to sell my electrolysis business. For the first five years I enjoyed many aspects of my business and learned a lot. The next five years were less challenging and less fun. The final four years I wanted out. But I worried about financial disaster. I was also concerned that I would never see any of my interesting clients again. When I finally did sell my business, I was so sick of it that living in a tent with no friends seemed like a better option. Being sick of your life *is* a great antidote for one's fears.

My family was not ruined financially, and the loss of my clientele was not as devastating as I had imagined. I think the more conscious fears of financial ruin and loss of clients obscured the deeper one of loss of self-identity. I had no idea what I was going to do next. I was surprised to feel so adrift, like being in a rudderless boat on the sea. I was no longer an expert at something, no longer knew what to expect from one minute to the next, even if those minutes were boring. I sometimes felt like a babe in the woods starting all over again, scared, awkward, stumbling.

I used my yoga experience, knowing that what I was going through was similar to putting my body into an unfamiliar and difficult yoga pose. I breathed through the anxiety as it surfaced, recognizing that I would eventually feel comfortable in my new life posture. It took time, but I had faith in the method.

The reward has been an exciting new focus in life.

Daily routine has a certain predictable comfort, but you can develop stiffness in the mind and body from it. When you finally let go you begin to see where you have narrowed your life, cut off possibilities.

Yoga discipline teaches the principles that make this kind of transition easier. It gives you a blueprint for handling the change. Starting over in a new relationship or a new profession or in anything is like learning a difficult new yoga posture. By acknowledging your fears, breathing into and releasing your anxieties, you gain flexibility and strength in your new life posture.

Improving your relationship with your body has the same elements. You will work through the pain of a constricted view of yourself. Before you gain the flexibility and strength in your new body image posture you may feel lost, angry, scared. But if you stick with the day-to-day process of what you are trying to accomplish, observing yourself, you redefine your self-image and create the life you want.

When you stretch the tight muscles of your body, you give yourself the opportunity to challenge the fears and anxieties that make them tight. In this way, changing the shape of your body changes you. You learn to relax in yoga poses, and the more relaxed you are, the more courage you have to create the life you want.

In order to progress in a life goal you need to challenge yourself by doing the hardest things that come to mind. A good yoga practice has the same element. Whatever the hardest element is, you incorporate some little piece of that element into your daily workout. You break your progress down into small-size, digestible bites.

Cultivating Daily Habit Exercises

Exercise 1

Each morning (forever) find a comfortable and quiet place (lying in your bed when you first get up is one suggestion).

Say to yourself, "I love the natural shape of my body."

Feel the love permeate every pore. At first you may not feel the emotion even if you say it. That's okay. Close your eyes and visualize the love as a sensation or a sound or a picture. For example, one friend visualized the love as a bright sunny light with a happy face in it. Eventually, if your desire is strong enough and you have a disciplined approach to achieving your goal, you will believe yourself.

Exercise 2

1. In the morning, think of something to do that is hard and challenging but makes you feel good about yourself.
2. Affirm that you intend that day to do it.
3. Visualize what steps you will take to do it.
4. Feel the emotions you will have when it is done.
5. Then do it.

Do this every day for a week.

Exercise 3

Pick something you would like to change in your life and document your efforts in a journal. Keep track of your progress in the journal every day for at least three months. At the end read your journal to see what you have learned about yourself. Pick something you feel you can be successful at.

If you practice yoga, pick a challenging pose to work with every day for three months. Write about your experience in the journal. See how working with that pose can give you insight into your ability to meet your goal.

Exercise 4

Pick a challenging area in your life you would like to change. Follow the same procedure as the first exercise and stick with your goal and your journal for however long it takes, one month, ten years, whatever.

CHAPTER 10

The Value
of Discipline

Journal Entry

I've been helping Neill in the gym, fetching the basketball as he practices his game. One day I noticed that he made about ten foul shots in a row. "I made twenty-five baskets in a row, last week," he bragged.

"Let me see you do it again, then," I said because I noticed that he had turned away from the foul line after missing his eleventh shot.

"Twenty-five in a row" has become a theme for the summer. That first day it took him a half hour to make the requisite number of shots. The next day was about the same. The third day he wouldn't leave practice until he made his twenty-five in a row, even though it took almost an hour and a half. Three days later, he couldn't sink twenty-five shots in a row to save his life.

Three weeks into our daily routine he began to tighten up as he approached the 20th shot, which caused him to miss at that point, over and over again. He had built up too much emotional attachment to the result. It took him a couple of weeks to work through his tightness of mind and attitude to the point where he was loose enough to get past his twentieth shot. He had come full *circle, in a way, being able to make 25 baskets in a row again, but with a new wisdom behind the ability.*

Neill's twenty-five-in-a-row summer is an introductory course on the essence of discipline. He learned that when you approach a goal with discipline you include work on what is the hardest for you to do, as well as doing what comes easily. Making inroads in the areas that you find the hardest to work on keeps you alert and your self-observation sharp, which is necessary in order to expand your boundaries.

At some point I have began to think of yoga as my spiritual practice. I'm not sure when or why. At lunch yesterday I said to Debra Ann that even without a spiritual element to it, the discipline of yoga is well worth all of the effort. Debra Ann replied that the discipline is the spiritual aspect of yoga.

I used to think that a disciplined life was rigid and boring, which is exactly how my undisciplined life was.

Commit yourself to a daily involvement in attaining your goal. When you approach a goal with daily discipline, you focus on what is in front of you right now. What you have now is your life and your breath. Without the breath there is no life. The breath is the defining aspect of life.

Journal Entry

Haven't noticed much progress in my yoga for months. Reviewed and concentrated on the basics today. Focused on finding the restricted areas of movement and bringing myself to the edge of discomfort. Relaxed and extended these spots in rhythm to deep, steady exhalations and inhalations.

The funny thing about progress is how unlike progress it feels on a daily basis. Every day of the practice you do the same thing. You bring yourself to the limit of movement; you observe and adjust yourself in the poses, using your breath to help you stay focused in the appropriate places. You breathe into the extension and release the tension. You do this every day, day after day after day.

And when you look back after two or three years of practice you realize how far you have come. Criteria that seemed so im-

portant in the early stages of your practice—how great or terrible you looked in the pose, or how you compared to other students in the class—become less important.

The meaning of the practice also changes. As you focus on the physical aspects other developments occur out of the corner of your eye. You become more centered within yourself and can more often acknowledge your strengths and weaknesses impartially. As your shape in the poses change, the shape of your body changes and the shape of your life changes, becoming more flexible, strong, and balanced.

Practice brings your attention and focus to exactly where you are now, physically, mentally, emotionally, and spiritually.

Discipline develops the courage and the power to create the lives we want. One reason for this is that to be disciplined, we have to pay attention to what is happening in the present. We spend a lot of time looking ahead into the future—with dread or anticipation—or back into the past—with regret or longing for what once was. Discipline keeps us focused in the present moment, where our lives are happening all around us. We have the power to effect change in our lives in the present

The future and past are all made up of present moments. Each present moment is the only living reality. Each present moment builds from the previous ones. The past is a compilation of all of the present moments that came before, and the future will be a compilation of all of the present moments that follow this one. The future will be shaped from present decisions and actions.

Coming back from one seminar, Bob asked me to make a statement about the future, which I did: If I sell my business I just know we'll end up living in a tent. He then asked me if the statement was true. Of course I said no because the future hadn't happened yet. He said any statement about the future has to be false for the same reason.

Facing a challenging task, an insurmountable mountain, or an abyss, or some other image your fears construct, may lurk to defeat you before you even start. One aspect of discipline is that you stay focused on your daily objectives and let your actions emanate from them. You focus on the reality of the present, not some illusion of possible defeating events that haven't yet occurred. You do this every day, day in and day out. Then, one day, you look around with surprise to see that the insurmountable mountain or the threatening abyss is behind you (I guess Len was right). And, you have accomplished a courageous thing.

Yoga practice can be your guidepost through the wilderness of transformation. It focuses your attention on what you are experiencing in the present moment. Its teachings are about equanimity. Equanimity means mental and emotional stability, presence of mind. If you can accept whatever outcome your decisions and actions bring (like maybe living in a tent is doable), then you have gained equanimity and have become wiser. Equanimity breeds courage. With equanimity, you are fearless in your choices. Fear obfuscates the wisdom within you.

You learn equanimity from yoga's meditative quality. While the practice has a sitting meditation pose, even the most physically demanding postures are meditative in nature. Meditation teaches you how to maintain presence of mind from moment to moment. You become more proficient at observing your thoughts with dispassion. You develop a habit that helps you become less attached to specific outcomes. In class the outcome may be how you look in or do a pose, but the technique carries over into the rest of your life. The more open you are to accept whatever outcomes emanate from your actions, the more relaxed you will be about what happens.

The more relaxed you are, the more courage you have.

In class one day, one of my yoga teachers quoted Mr. Iyengar (author of *Light on Yoga* and one of the most widely read and influential yogis) as saying that balance is falling over equally in all directions. Can you see how balance would make all outcomes of your decisions equally okay?

An article in *Yoga Journal* says that the yogi warrior must harness the wild movements of the mind and emotions. These are what create turmoil in our lives and keep us from acting from our balanced centers. Warrior Pose helps us to locate our center of gravity and develop balance.

Warrior Pose Exercise

(This is one of several variations.)

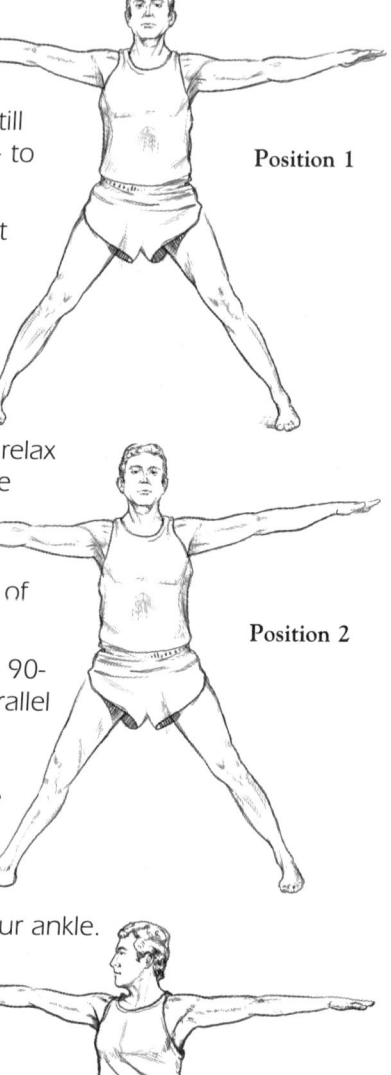

1. Stand with your feet together in Mountain Pose.

2. Step to the right so your feet are still parallel to each other and about 4 to 4½ feet apart.

3. Raise your arms to shoulder height (see position 1).

Position 1

4. Point your right foot toward the wall in front of it and turn your left foot in at about a 30-degree angle (see position 2).

5. Breathe deeply and evenly as you relax your sacrum and sink your tailbone neutrally to the floor.

6. Elongate your spine. Lengthen your arms starting from the center of your body outward.

Position 2

7. Bend your right knee until it is at a 90-degree angle and your thigh is parallel to the floor as you can make it. As you bend imagine someone holding your left hand back by the tips of your fingers. This will help keep your torso straight and centered over your hips. Do not extend your bent knee past your ankle.

8. Turn your head and look out over your extended right arm with a soft and relaxed gaze (see position 3).

Position 3

9. Do you feel centered and strong in the pose? Breathe deeply and evenly for five breaths.

10. Come back up to position 2.

11. Repeat the pose to the opposite side, starting with step 4 and ending with step 9.

12. Step your feet together and stand quietly in Mountain Pose for a moment.

Journal Entry

Debra Ann used lots of props in yoga class today. One was a killer. Yoga practice is supposed to focus your attention on what you are doing now. If your mind has inadvertently strayed from the present, there is no substitute for a killer-prop to bring it back.

I positioned myself on the prop. Ouch. I felt the unforgiving wood dig into my tailbone and sacrum. The prop had grown barbs, or so it felt.

"You must breathe and relax into the props," Debra Ann says, "take the hint from what they are trying to teach you." They show you where you need to relax and let go, where you need to get stronger and bring more energy. They teach you balance and equanimity in a pose.

Okay.

One reason I put off starting yoga classes for so long was that I didn't feel it would give me the aerobic workout I was getting in classes at the gym. Isabelle, my first teacher, gave very gentle classes, which is what I needed to start.

However, when I started taking classes with Debra Ann, even though I was lifting weights and jogging, I found myself crawling from one pose to the next midway through. The stiffer you are, the more aerobic the session feels. Strength includes balance and flexibility.

A student in another class had the same misconception about yoga. During class one day she told Emma, our teacher, she had always thought yoga classes were not aerobic enough. One session, which included a more advanced version of Sun Salutation, revised that notion.

The object of yoga poses on a daily basis is not to do a perfect pose. What you can and cannot do varies from session to session. What it teaches you is how to be present and patient with your body exactly where it is in the moment. Paying attention and using your breath is essential.

It is generally acknowledged that deep, slow breathing calms anxiety. Breathing evenly and calmly is hard to remember when you feel anxious or afraid. Your daily practice with the edge trains you to remember. Using focused breathing in yoga poses in the calm and disciplined setting of a class or at home, eventually carries over into everyday life. In time you learn how to breathe more easily through all of life's challenges.

I have been told repeatedly how important the breath is in yoga postures. By focusing on steady rhythmic breathing, you focus your attention on your body and mind in the present, in the pose.

The natural shape of your body changes in a rhythm similar to that which you observe with your breath. Just as one breath cycle is different from the previous one, so is each state of your natural body different from the previous one. As you learn to calmly let go from one breath to the next, you learn to live peacefully in the present state of your body from one moment to the next.

Your body constantly changes. It is, in a way, a process rather than a solid object. Therefore, revising a body image is an ongoing process. Your ability to know when you need to make an adjustment in your life is influenced greatly by your ability to observe yourself dispassionately at times. You know how much easier it is to see what others need to do and so much harder to know what you need to do. Fear pulls a veil over one's eyes.

You don't have to figure everything out mentally first. You don't need to dig up whatever obscure reasons from the past are twisting your life out of shape so that then, theoretically, you could fix it and comfortably move on. Fear isn't that accommodating. It does not step aside once you have an intellectual understanding of what is going on. Like the title of a popular book by Susan Jeffers says, you need to *Feel the Fear and Do It Anyway*. When you do it anyway, you don't have to search hard for the reasons that keep you back; they tend to surface pretty quickly.

Finding the Promised Land, happiness, and comfort with your natural shape, involves dealing with fear and judgment. Judgment about the worthiness of yourself and others. Fear of how things will look when you are different. Fear of being different. However, the journey is well worth it.

The daily practice of yoga changes your life in increments that may seem minuscule, like the grains of sand that together make up a beach. You improve your self-image by staying focused on your goal and working every day to achieve it.

Breath Exercise

1. Sit on a mat or carpet on the floor.

2. Place your hands on either side of your hips (see position 1).

Position 1

3. Search for your tailbone with your mind.

4. Starting from your tailbone, roll your torso down one vertebra at a time until your head is relaxed on the floor.

5. Extend your right leg out.

6. Extend your left leg out.

7. You should now be supine on the floor (see position 2).

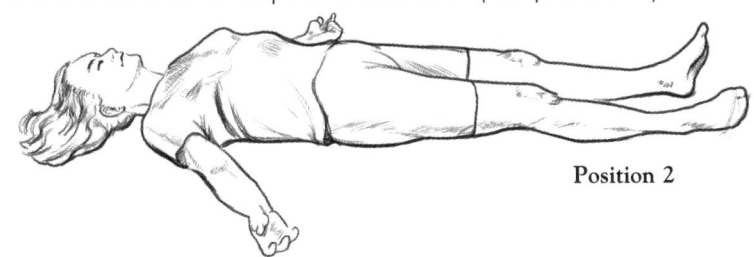

Position 2

8. Breathe normally in this position for five minutes.

9. Place your hands on your stomach, your thumbs resting lightly on your navel (see position 3).

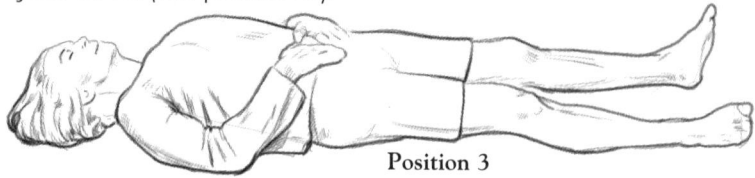

Position 3

10. Breathe deeply into the touch of your hands on your stomach. You should feel your hands move as your stomach expands. Breathe like this for three minutes.

11. Place your hands on your rib cage so that your pinkies align with the bottom of your ribs (see position 4).

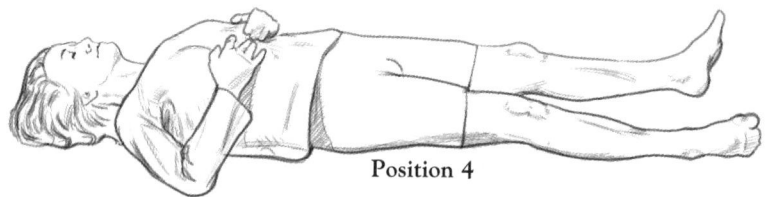

Position 4

12. Breathe into the touch of your hands on your rib cage. You should feel your fingers move as your rib cage expands.

13. Breathe like this for three minutes.

14. Place your hands on your upper rib cage (see position 5).

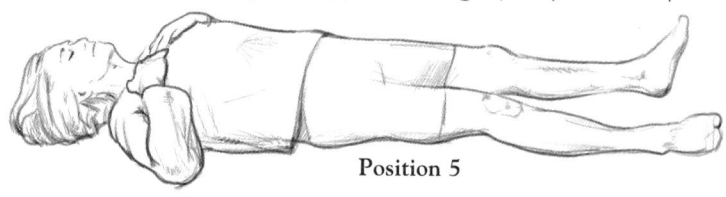

Position 5

15. Breathe into the touch of your hands. You should feel your fingers move as your upper rib cage expands.

16. Breathe like this for three minutes.

17. Bring your arms back to your sides. Roll to one side and gently sit up.

CHAPTER 11

The Promised Land in Sight

Bob and I met Zhu, our qi gong instructor, in the summer of 1998. He came from China and lived in our house his first summer in America. Qi gong means "energy work" and its cultivation of internal energy is the basis of the power of the Chinese martial arts.

The basic form of qi gong Zhu teaches is standing meditation. The fundamental principles of qi gong and yoga are the same. Both practices develop a strong, flexible body and cultivate life force energy, known as qi (pronounced "chee") in the Chinese system and prana in the Indian yoga system.

Zhu, like Debra Ann, has X-ray vision into the energy flow of the body.

Journal Entry

"Tuck your pelvis," says Zhu, as he observes me in standing meditation. I need to tuck my pelvis so that it does not tilt forward, spilling the imaginary liquid it is holding onto the floor. What a struggle—I tuck, after several minutes my pelvis tilts, I tuck, it stubbornly tilts.

Today I was able to pinpoint the moment and bodily location when and where my pelvis begins to tilt forward. I focused on that precise juncture, heading off the tilt at the pass. Three areas of my body were highlighted as I did this. The muscles in my upper back

117

ached as they were forced to maintain an unfamiliar stretch, my ankles felt pressured to bend more deeply, and the soles of my feet were hot and angry as they, too, were stretched to their limit.

Standing meditation often highlights groups of body areas at one time. When one part of the body is out of alignment, other parts of the body adjust to compensate for the distortion. Together they form an unaligned equilibrium. Standing meditation transforms the unaligned equilibrium into a centered equilibrium.

All parts of my body are interrelated. My stomach and waist are an integral part of the rest of my body and their natural shape and size fit in with my body as a whole. The idea of exchanging parts of my body by putting it on a frame seems silly now, as it always was, except for the emotional anguish that accompanied the notion. The flat stomach and tiny waist of my dreams do not fit in with the overall shape of the rest of my body.

An example of an unaligned equilibrium comes from the book *Somatics* by Thomas Hanna. Suppose, Hanna says, an injury occurs to one side of the body that causes the muscles of the pelvis and lumbar spine to contract more tightly on one side. In order to remain upright the body's equilibrium system will adjust, pulling the head and upper trunk to the opposite side to counterbalance the lower tilt. The body now has a new upright equilibrium comprised of the unaligned balance of the upper and lower halves of the body.

Body alignment, Mr. Hanna says, gets distorted not only from physical trauma but also from habitual stress, as mentioned earlier. Bodily changes—stooped shoulders, chronically contracted abdominal muscles and hamstrings, swayback posture, wrinkled brows to name a few—which are various combinations of the effects of the red light and green light reflexes, create the familiar postures of old age. All of these postural problems result in blocked energy flow in the body.

Our Western point of view does not focus on activities that develop the body as a whole entity, made up not only of its parts, but of its mind as well. We work on our bodies. We work on our minds. We

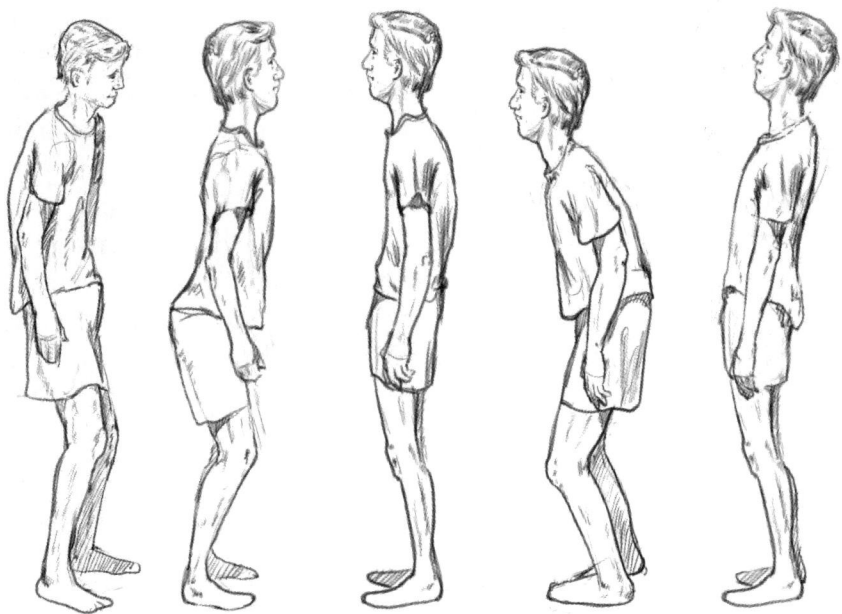

The familiar postures of old age.

work on our emotions. We recognize the connections between the three but we do not engage in activities that cultivate the connections.

A TV ad for a chain health club displays closeups of fabulous abs, chests, breasts, and thighs. The only pictures of whole people are in the fuzzy recesses of the background. Besides toned and strong muscles, your body needs good energy flow.

The energy flow of a body with postural unalignment is noticeably diminished. One chiropractor has said that our bodies expend about 85 percent of their energy working to stay upright in the field of gravity. You have to work harder to keep your upright posture against the flow of gravity if your body is out of alignment. Ida Rolf in her book *Ida Rolf Talks About Rolfing and Physical Reality* says to let gravity nourish you. The way you can get gravity to be more of a friend is to bring your body back into postural alignment. You can tell the difference when it is, it feels and moves more lightly.

I recently observed a woman with the toned muscles of someone who works out in the gym. She would easily have met the qualifications for fabulous arms and thighs on the TV ad, but she had no connected energy flow through her spine. She moved somewhat like a disjointed marionette.

The difference between workouts in the gym and yoga and qi gong is that the latter practices cultivate the harmony of mind and body working together on a single task. They improve the flow of energy through the body by releasing energy blockages like the ones I have mentioned. Spinning is one example of a workout in which mind and body are often focused on different activities. People pedal bicycle wheels while the rest of their attention is focused on watching television or reading a newspaper.

Yoga and qi gong train your whole body and mind to work together in every pose, which is how they differ from most ordinary exercise. The natural shape of your body evolves from this training.

Tree Pose Exercise

Good energy flow in alignment with gravity creates flexibility, strength, and balance. When your posture is aligned with gravity, you have good balance.

The following pose is called Tree Pose.

1. Stand with your feet together, your big toes touching each other (see position 1).
2. Relax your feet completely on the floor.
3. Lift your ankles and lengthen your legs from your ankles, up through your calves and shins and thighs.

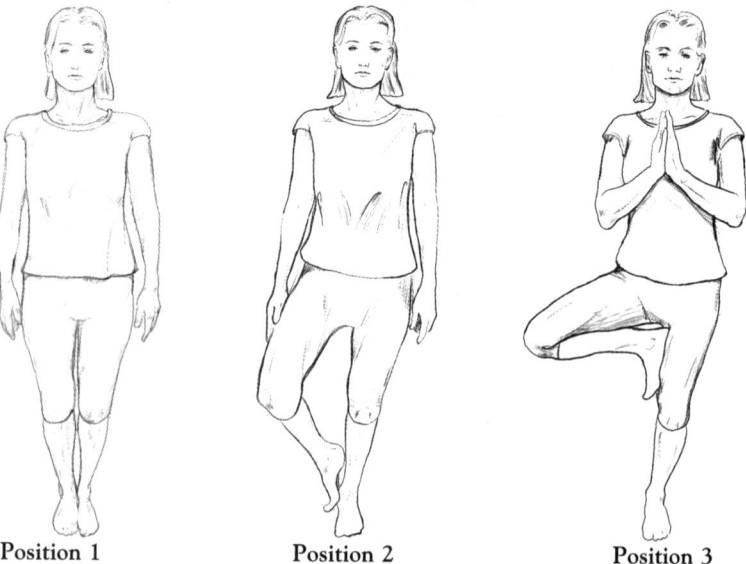

Position 1   Position 2   Position 3

4. Lift up your kneecaps to firm your thighs.

5. Lengthen your spine from the tailbone up and feel the length extend through the crown of your head.

6. Relax and widen your shoulders.

7. Turn your right foot out (see position 2).

8. Lift your foot and place it against your left thigh.

9. Bring your hands together (see position 3).

   If you are not flexible enough to place your foot in this position, place it lower on your leg.

10. Stand like this for forty seconds.

11. Repeat on the opposite side.

Journal Entry

Downward-Facing Dog pose made me feel twisted for a very long time. I don't look twisted to the casual eye, but I am. My chiropractor pointed out that my hips are rotated to the right instead of facing forward. The rest of my body has readjusted itself to compensate. My head and neck are twisted to the left so that I can look straight ahead.

Without a point of reference, I didn't know I was crooked. My crooked posture felt straight to me. Aligning myself in yoga created that point of reference. My body was unaligned in so many different ways—besides my hips, my shoulders were scrunched up, my hamstrings were as tight as strung catgut—the list seemed endless. Every new pose seemed to uncover a new imbalance.

What good is a 21-inch waist on a crooked body?

Yoga has reshaped my body and changed my posture. My legs and spine are straighter. My hips are less twisted. My shoulders are more relaxed and broader. I walk with a more confident gait and I dance more rhythmically.

Sometimes when I follow the points of awareness in a yoga posture I can sense a new way of arranging my body in space before I can actually do it. It is as if my mind conceives the next step in my body's transformation before the physical change occurs; like an artist's preconception of a new work.

In this manner a new sense of my stomach is developing; it flits within the borders of my awareness briefly and then disappears, a ghostly reality that has not yet taken substantive form, a preliminary mind-sketch that is not yet filled with color and depth.

The evolving shape of my stomach is not the super-flat stomach of my ideal body image, nor is it the tight, dense, round stomach I have had for the past twenty years. My new stomach is round, but smaller and softer; it reminds me of my ten-year-old stomach. A more natural shape.

My evolving body shape is superior to the ideal body I thought I wanted.

When your body shape gets distorted from the stresses of life over the years, you have no frame of reference to remind you of how you once were. Yoga practice provides that frame of reference. When a yoga teacher points out what you need to do to improve a pose, she is showing you how to return your body to its more natural state.

As dead zones come to life when your body opens up, your body starts to provide you with an expanded frame of reference. As new areas open up in what used to be dead zones they provide the opening for further expansion and greater alignment in a bootstrap type of process.

Journal Entry

Won the 3.0 division of the Gates Tennis Ladder. I have my first trophy ever. I am a much better tennis player even though I haven't taken lessons in years. I spent the whole summer working on my game, observing my play with the practiced eye of a yogini.

The biggest improvement in my game is my ability to run down balls as they come over the net. My feet are more flexible and mobile and I am much faster on the court. I am in love with my new feet.

The second most noticeable improvement is my ability to focus on and achieve a goal.

Journal Entry

In my next life, if I have a next life, I want to be an Olympic rhythmic gymnast. For the past two weeks, late at night when everyone else is asleep, I have been watching the tapes I made of the Olympic competition. The tapes have temporarily replaced my customary late night mystery novel.

I find the gymnasts' graceful, incredibly flexible, and strong movements mesmerizing and mysterious. I play one sequence over and over again, in real time, then in slow motion. Ukrainian gymnast Yelena Vitrishenko starts her movement seated between her bent legs. She propels herself up, onto her toes, her back arching so that her head practically touches the backs of her knees. Like this:

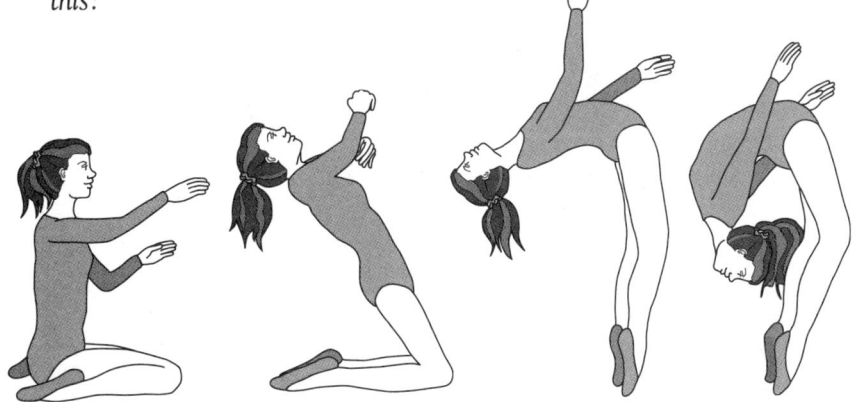

How does she do this? How come her ankles don't break in two? I played the tape for Bob and Neill.

"She must use the muscles in her thighs" Neill theorized.

"I don't think so," I said, remembering that Zhu says movement starts in the tailbone.

She was not using the muscles of her legs; she was propelling herself up in space with the strength and movement of her spine. Her body followed the movement of her spine. She seemed weightless.

No, I will not fabricate a new ideal body image. I will not envision wrapping my leg like a shawl around my shoulders, as Yana Batryshina did.

Bob has noticed the beautiful curving shape of the neck and upper backs of the gymnasts who perform on the balance beams and other apparatus; it follows the spine's natural curve.

(Note: Rhythmic gymnasts, not to be confused with the gymnasts who perform on apparatus, compete with dancelike floor routines using ribbons and balls and ropes as props. The sequence I describe is from the 1998 Summer Olympics.)

You don't have to be a 110-pound (or less) gymnast in order to move with weightless grace. When heavyweight wrestler Rulon Gardner won his gold medal in an upset at the 2000 Summer Olympics he did a cartwheel of joy. His 286-pound body moved with the same kind of weightless grace.

I discovered how much my spine had deteriorated when I visited a chiropractor after my most recent car accident. The chiropractor took X-rays of my thoracic spine.

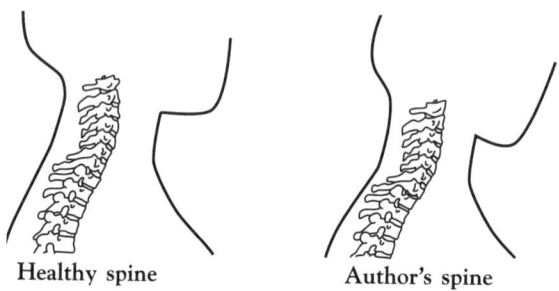

Healthy spine   Author's spine

After leaving the chiropractor's office, I was confused for some time. With my spine thrust forward like the X-ray showed, it seemed to me that its position inside my head must have shifted and that it was somehow closer to my mouth. That notion seemed weird. I didn't feel my spine tickling the back of my teeth.

My confusion was cleared up during one of my first qi gong classes. Zhu said, "First we work on hips, then we get to neck later." I wondered how he knew about my neck.

I later examined the profile of my neck in the mirror and understood how Zhu knew about my neck. In the mirror I saw that my spine had not shifted closer to my mouth. My neck was thrust forward and my head was scrunched down. I had pictured my spine closer to my mouth because my mental image was of my head still sitting straight over my shoulders. My altered sense of straight had escaped my notice because it had taken place over many years.

I stretched my neck and adjusted the tilt of my head to smooth out the kink in the curve of my spine. In this position I could feel the tight muscles in my upper back and sternum being pulled as well as a tugging in my diaphragm and groin. Neill measured me in this adjusted posture and I was ½ inch taller than my current height.

With regret, I dropped my head back to its now habitual position. The shift in the position of my head is one reason why I am more than an inch shorter than I used to be.

The deterioration in my spine probably started very young. When I was seventeen, I suffered severe whiplash in a car accident and I have been in a total of three accidents. In each accident, the car behind me smashed into and shoved my car forward.

I imagine a lifetime struggle being a part of the accident, the cosmic interaction as follows:

Me (daydreaming): "One day I'm really going to show the world what I can do...when I've got it all together...when I have the money...when the time is right..."

Cosmos (in the form of a distracted driver behind me): "For God's sake, Barbara, just do it."

The Olympic athletes inspired me because with my experience of yoga, I comprehend a way to acquire a lot of the flexibility and body control that they have, within my own body. Along the way I will regain whatever I can of the health of my spine.

Will I ever have a completely healthy, normal spine again? Zhu thinks I will.

He expects that my head will again sit straight on my shoulders, like it was meant to do. I have already made great progress. While my spine is not yet straight, it is healthier than it was. Before yoga my neck was unrelentingly sore and stiff. Daily practice has taken away the soreness and restored a large amount of mobility.

There are many stories about how the body can be repaired through yoga practice.

Bikram Choudhury, author of *Bikram's Beginning Yoga Class* mentioned earlier, is the founder of an international school of yoga. The beginning pages of the book describe how he had won the National Yoga Contest of India for three years. At seventeen his knee was injured and European doctors predicted that he would never walk again. He had himself carried back to his teacher and after six months of yoga his knee was healed.

The health of your body is greatly improved with good posture. So are its shape and grace. Good posture comes from a healthy spine.

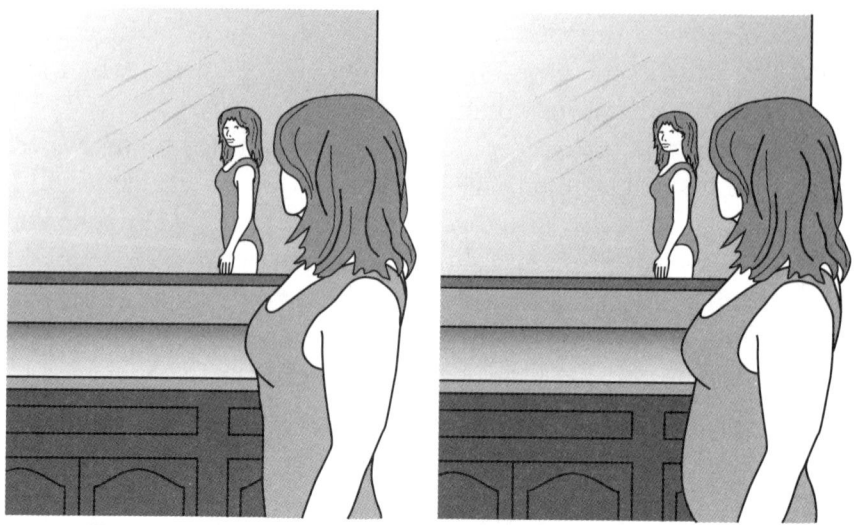

You can really tell how the perceived shape of my stomach changes.

Postural Exercises

Exercise 1

1. In a full-length mirror, stand so you can observe your profile.

2. Adjust your posture by following the instructions for Mountain Pose on pages 77 and 78. How does your posture in Mountain Pose compare to how you first looked in the mirror?

3. Now adjust your posture so that your shoulders are as stooped as you can make them.

4. Play around with other, in-between postures. Notice how these postures affect the overall shape of the different parts of your body.

Exercise 2

1. Spinal twists help to elongate and strengthen the spine.

2. Sit in a comfortable, armless chair with your feet flat on the floor and to one side of the chair (see position 1).

3. Place your hands on each side of the chair.

4. Sit up tall.

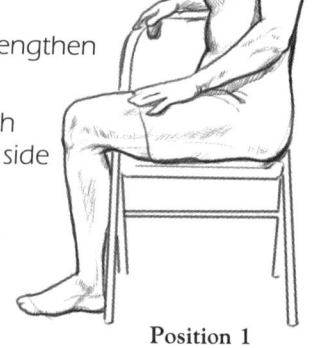

Position 1

126

5. Extend the crown of your head toward the ceiling.

6. Sink your tailbone into the chair.

7. Relax your shoulders.

8. Take a few deep breaths and relax all over.

9. Inhale deeply, lengthen your spine, and on the exhalation twist to your right from your tailbone up through the crown of your head. Use your hands on the chair to maintain your upright posture as you twist.

10. Look as far to the right as you can (see position 2).

11. Inhale deeply again, lengthen your spine more, and on the exhalation deepen the twist. Look farther to the right.

Position 2

12. Repeat step 11 one more time.

13. Release the twist. Sit on the chair with your legs over the opposite side.

14. Repeat the exercise twisting to your left.

Exercise 3

During the day, whenever you remember, extend the crown of your head toward the ceiling and sink your tailbone to the floor. Notice how the different areas of your body feel when you do this.

Journal Entry

Bob and I went to see a play last week. A man sat down in front of me. He wasn't that tall, but he sat very straight. I had to straighten up my normal slouch in order to see over his head. After a while I began to pay attention to his posture. He sat straight, but not ramrod straight. I sensed no tension in his posture; he exuded physical ease and comfort. He sat straight and at ease at the same time. I had never seen anyone sit like that.

I wondered if he practiced yoga, or maybe some form of martial art. He must have been in his thirties. To get to that age with *such intact posture, could it be done without the help of some regular practice? If I weren't so shy I would have tapped him on the shoulder and asked him what he did. What would it feel like to have his kind of posture? What I would never have the courage to ask him: Excuse me sir, could I borrow your spine for a little while?*

A degenerating disc, which is what I have in my neck, causes loss of height with age. I heard on the radio that there is a formula for the average loss of height with age. One former client dismissed my concern: "Everyone has degenerating discs when they get older," he said.

I don't think so, even though degenerative discs are probably very common with age. My friend Lynn is three months older than I and should therefore be at least a micromillimeter shorter than I am but she is not. She is still 5 feet 4½ inches tall, which is what we both were when we met eighteen years ago. I don't think she has any degenerating discs. She is fifty-one years old and still the same height she was when she was thirty-three. Lynn and I have probably together lost the average amount of height.

Without yoga practice my shrinkage would probably continue at an alarming rate. When I took my father in for his last physical and the nurse asked his height, we both paused, confused about what to put down. My father used to be 6 feet tall, but now he and I look each other in the eye. A lot of the length of his upper spine is curved over and his legs stay bent all of the time.

With yoga practice I have regained some of my lost height in the past couple of years. Neill and I take turns measuring each other periodically. He is hoping to break through the 6-foot barrier. I am hoping to get back to 5 feet 4½ . He is growing taller and I am straightening out.

The philosophies of both yoga and qi gong teach that a healthy spine is important for good health and aging gracefully.

The red light and green light reflexes combine to form the typical postures of old age (see page 121). You can see how the reaction to stress over the period of a lifetime shortens your body and distorts your spine. Compare this with the picture of the elderly qi gong master (page 44).

Sadie Delany on yoga: "I started doing yoga exercises with Mama about forty years ago. Mama was starting to shrink up and get bent down, and I started exercising with her to straighten her up again....I kept doing my yoga exercises, even after Mama died. Well, when Bessie turned eighty she decided that I looked better than her. So she decided she would start doing yoga, too."

Teachers of both yoga and qi gong talk about moving the spine one vertebra at a time. A healthy spine can do this.

Healthy Spine Exercises

(The following exercises help to create healthy, flexible spines.)

Exercise 1

Qi gong spinal roll:

1. Stand with your feet hip distance apart and parallel to each other (see position 1).

2. Lengthen your spine. Imagine a tail extending from your tailbone to the floor.

3. Slowly raise your hands in front of your chest. Relax your elbows and shoulders down (see position 2).

4. Raise your elbows shoulder level.

5. Relax your elbows and wrists. One way to do this is to imagine they have small weights resting on them.

6. Keeping your elbows slightly bent, extend your forearms in front of you (see position 3).

7. Relax from your shoulders to your elbows. Then relax from your elbows to the tips of your fingers.

8. Bend forward, keeping your back straight. Imagine someone pulling your fingers gently away from you (see position 4).

9. Let your spinal column fall forward, one vertebra at a time, keeping your back straight for as long as possible. When you can no longer keep your back straight without bending your knees let it curve and round forward all the way.

10. Extend the crown of your head toward the floor.

11. To come back up, roll your spine up. Start from the tailbone, one vertebra at a time. If your spine has good flexibility, you will be able to feel and move each separate vertebra in this exercise (see position 5).

If you suddenly fall forward in a chunk without control at a certain point, then that is where you need to work on the health of your spine.

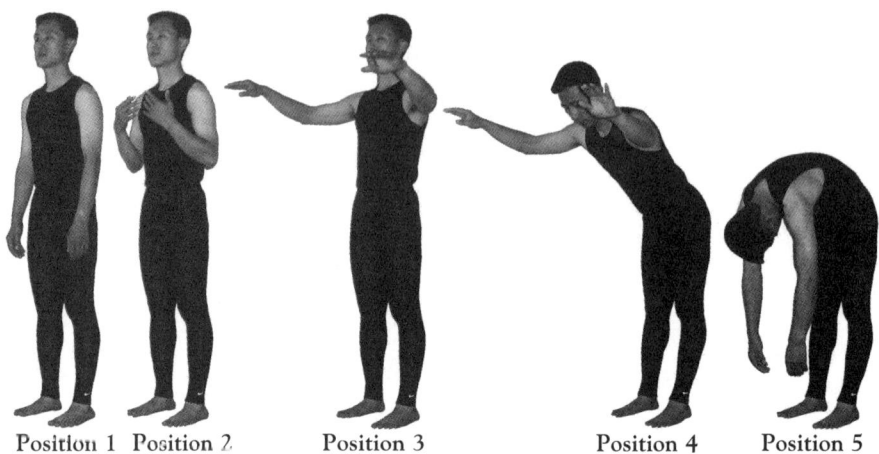

Position 1 Position 2 Position 3 Position 4 Position 5

Exercise 2
Yoga Cat Stretch:

1. Place your hands and knees on the flc Your hands should be directly under your shoulders and your knees directly under your hips, as pictured (see position 1).

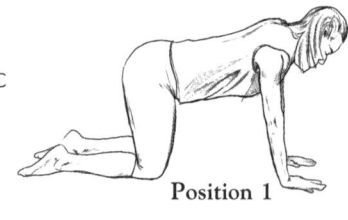

Position 1

2. Breathe normally for several moment without altering your breath's rhythm

3. Lengthen your breath by breathing deeply into the belly and up into the chest for a minute or so.

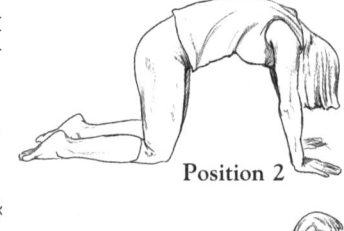

Position 2

4. On an inhalation curl your back, mak front of your body concave (see posit

5. On the next exhalation do the oppos making your back concave (see posit

6. Repeat steps 4 and 5 for ten cycles, minimum.

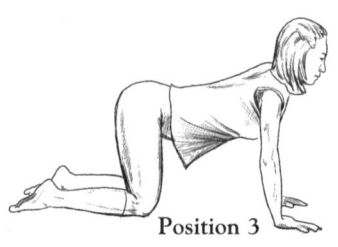

Position 3

Exercise 3

Yoga Cobra Pose:

1. You can use a yoga mat or lie down on a carpeted floor for this pose.

2. Lie prone on the floor.

3. Put your hands on the floor along the sides of your body so that the tips of your fingers are aligned with the top of your shoulders.

4. Spread your fingers wide and relax your palms. Make sure that your middle fingers point directly forward.

5. Bring your legs together (see position 1).

6. On an exhalation relax your thighs away from your hips along their length on the floor.

7. On the next exhalation relax your sacrum and let your tailbone sink toward the floor. (As you follow this instruction you will feel a tightening in your buttocks.)

8. On the next exhalation sink your navel into the floor and feel your whole body expand in the pose.

Position 1

9. On an inhalation look up and curl your spine up from the floor, letting the crown of your head reach for the ceiling. Do not lift yourself up using your arms; your hands on the floor are only to balance you in the pose (see position 2).

Position 2

10. Lift your hands slightly off the floor (see position 3).

11. Breathe deeply and evenly, continuing to lengthen your spine for thirty seconds.

Position 3

12. Slowly lower your head back down to the floor.

13. Repeat the pose a second time.

Journal Entry

*As I focused on the points of awareness for Plow Pose to-
day—relaxing my sternum, lifting up my hips by extending the
lumbar and sacrum—I felt as if my legs and back were being
supported by a new energy flow. That region of my body felt ex-
traordinary, as if it had developed a new life of its own.*

*Forward Bend is so different now, too. Relaxed in the pose, I
can move my mind along the bones of my legs and soften and
extend them; I can consciously feel and widen different sections of
my back.*

When you practice yoga your mind/body awareness grows. You
no longer feel like an inept juggler in the poses. The different parts
of your body perform like actors in a play who have all learned their
roles well. When all of the actors perform their roles in harmony the
whole is a cohesive play. A play is much more than the sum of the
actors saying their lines, just as a sentence is more than the sum of its
words.

Remember how you connected the numbered dots as a child in
order to reveal the picture of an animal? When you connect the
points of awareness you have focused on repeatedly over years and
years of practice, a larger, integrated picture of your body emerges.
With awareness present everywhere in your body the energy flow
you create is more than the sum of the parts. The change within you
can feel as dramatic as Pinocchio metamorphosing from a wooden
puppet into a person.

With complete mind/body connection you are in control of your
body and understand it; you appreciate and respect it immensely.

Journal Entry

*I saw a TV program that featured the most flexible man, ac-
cording to The Guinness Book of World Records. He could turn
his legs in his sockets so that his knees faced backward when he
walked. Is there such a thing as being too flexible?*

*One of the rhythmic gymnasts on my tape overextended her
body in her dance routines; she was so flexible her form lacked
crispness, it looked soggy, like a cooked noodle. There is a balance*

point between tight and loose, and if you go over either way, you lose awareness, strength, and form.

I remember one example from my Phoenix Rising Yoga Therapy training. Michael Lee was demonstrating how to assist in a yoga posture in which the recipient of the technique is lying supine on the floor. One leg is lifted straight up and brought down along that side of the body, bringing it to the floor, if possible, and then up toward the head. He demonstrated this on someone who was as loose as a rag doll. She looked as if she could probably have moved her leg 360 degrees around her body if her head weren't in the way.

Most of the time the assisting person helps the recipient to extend the posture as far as she can, into the edge. For this woman, Mr. Lee stopped with her leg halfway up to her head. The student squirmed with discomfort and then started to cry. I remember this so well, because I had inadvertently achieved the same result. I had been partnered with someone who was just as flexible earlier that day. I had not exerted enough pressure to bring my partner to her edge because I had been afraid of hurting her. She kept asking for more pressure but I demurred. She seemed really angry with me at the end.

A friend of mine has this kind of flexibility in her lower legs. It seems to me that our bodies match our habits. She handles things that bother her in a way that reminds me of the Phoenix Rising Therapy session. She lets people push and push as she mentally and emotionally withdraws from the pressure. She thins the pressure out until she can completely ignore the problem. Echoing her mental/emotional process, her lower body is overly lax. I stew over a problem, making it dense and thick in my body and mind. My whole body is overly contracted.

Being too flexible in an area is not a problem I have had to deal with much. Bob remembers being flexible as a child; I don't. Yet I was flexible, once. I have pictures from childhood to prove it. In one photograph I am sitting under a Christmas tree, my legs spread out straight in front of me in a pose that has only now, after more than ten years of yoga, begun to feel okay.

As I have worked on my body over the years, I have released old traumas and habitual patterns of stress. I wondered if I have anything happy stored in my body. I do, only the happy parts do not retain chronic stress and anxiety. They are a part of my body's natural shape.

One day, as Zhu explained the benefits of qi gong he said that qi gong brings your body back to its natural state, like when you were a baby. "The natural body shape." The phrase encapsulates the changes that have taken place in my body.

Yoga does the same thing; it helps you regain your natural body shape. I don't know whether we even have our most natural shapes as babies. Sometimes I think the natural body shape goes beyond that because babies have within them the seeds of the crooked shapes they will deteriorate into.

I recently watched a middle school basketball team (teenage boys) stretch before a game. Most of them were already tight in their hips and legs. When they stretched out over spread legs on the floor, they looked like little hunchbacks. I think yoga and qi gong can return us to a state that may be more natural than the one in which we were born. I guess you could consider this an evolution of the soul.

What does your natural body shape look like? Your natural body shape is uniquely yours. My natural body shape is uniquely mine. There can never be media images that are exactly like either one. Your natural body shape will not appear in a magazine unless you are being photographed for the picture. Your natural body shape is made up of your mind/body/emotions and spirit; it is emotional and thoughtful as much as it is a physical shape. It is centered and peaceful.

Your natural body shape is a synergistic blend of mind/body/emotions and spirit.

Part III

The Promised Land

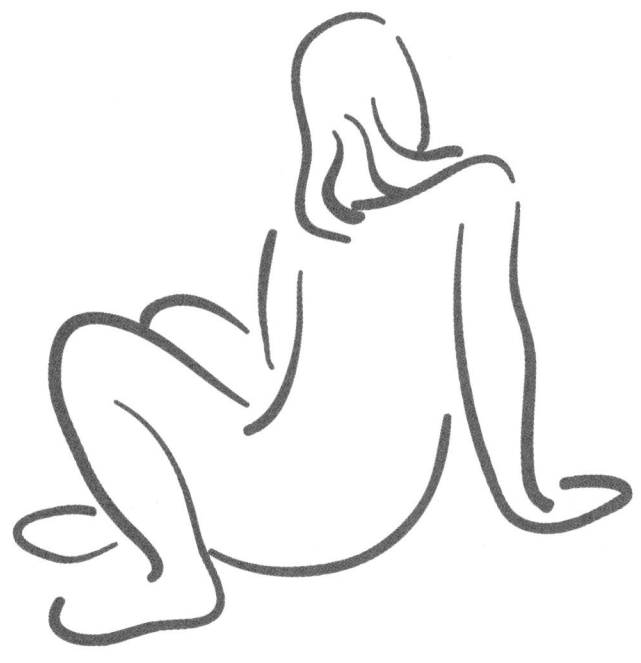

CHAPTER 12

Cultivating Your Natural Body Shape

Your Natural Body Shape is a work of art that emerges in a process similar to how Michelangelo created the Pieta. Michelangelo was asked how he knew what part of the original stone to chip away. He said that he chipped away everything that was not the Pieta. What remained became his masterpiece.

Your natural body shape is an expression of your natural self. Chronic anxiety, fear, and anger distort the natural shape of your body. Yoga and qi gong are the chisels that return it to its natural shape. They help you to discover or rediscover the connection between the energy patterns of your mind, the energy patterns of your emotions, and the energy patterns of your body. Your natural body shape is what remains after you chip away your deepest held fears, resentments, insecurities, and judgments.

Your natural body shape is made up of *your* waist, *your* hips, *your* thighs, and *your* face. And all other parts that are uniquely yours. When you uncover your own masterpiece you accept and find peace with a shape that was naturally yours all along.

Cultivating your natural body shape has spectacular rewards.

Journal Entry

Bob told me that one of his acquaintances from the gym had joked about seeing Neill fooling around with a pretty young girl instead of concentrating on basketball. Bob was confused at first. Then, putting two and two together, he realized that the "pretty young girl" had to be me.

For a while I indulged in some delicious speculation. I tried to imagine this man's vantage point. He might have peeked in from the entrance door to the basketball court, a distance of three-quarters of the court. Or he might have looked down from the jogging track, which rings the court from about 10 feet above. He probably only glanced at us. Still, to be mistaken for a contemporary of my teenage son really made my day. After all, I am fifty years old.

Last week the parents of one of Neill's friends made a similar mistake. Neill had driven me to their house and in the dim light of their garage both parents mistook me for a high school student.

I know I am in good physical shape because I watch my diet and exercise but to be mistaken for more than 30 years younger from a distance, by people who are not blind or senile, has to be credited to my years of practicing yoga and qi gong.

And to Charlie, hair stylist extraordinaire, who colors my gray with highlights that could fool Mother Nature. (I hope she doesn't hear this and get mad.)

Part of the youthful aura brought about by yoga and qi gong practice comes from the physical benefits. Your spine becomes straighter and more flexible. Your muscles return to the toned, elongated shape of youth. Your hips, shoulders, and knees regain lost mobility. Remember the flexibility and strength of the qi gong master on page 44?

The other aspects of the youthful aura brought about by yoga and qi gong practice come from training your mind to remain calm and open to new possibilities; and to learning emotional equanimity—which means becoming less attached to the outcome of events. A calm mind and emotional stability are tools for handling life more easily, creating less stress and slowing down physical aging.

The natural curve of the spine looks like this:

The natural state of the muscles is relaxed, toned, balanced.

The natural state of the emotions is the joy and peace that come from living in the present and not being attached to the outcome of events.

The natural state of the mind is meditative—quiet and calm.

The natural state of the spirit is the calm and courageousness that come from discipline.

You get great body image rewards from the cultivation of your natural body shape.

Another reward that comes from developing your natural body shape is the extra energy available for your life.

Journal Entry

I used to hang upside down using special boots attached to a bar in order to stretch my spine. The twists and stretches in yoga and qi gong stretch my spine, too. My spine is more flexible now than it was twenty years ago. Young people move differently than old people because their spines are straighter and more flexible.

Coming home from a Colorado University basketball game with Neill (he asked me along because none of his friends wanted to go), I watched a woman walking ahead of me as we left the game. From the back she looked fit and trim. But without seeing her face I knew she was middle-aged. Her walk gave her away. I have noticed this kind of walk in other women my age and older. We lose our range of motion in our hip joints and so to compensate we walk with smaller, scurrying steps. Our hips move in a chunk, swaying from side to side like a small pendulum.

As people get older they chunk up. Their shoulders become one chunk, their hips another, their upper back another, and their ankles yet another. Joints that once moved freely get stuck, like the rusted out gears of a machine that hasn't been oiled properly.

The natural body is like a machine that has been oiled and serviced regularly. It ages more slowly and gracefully.

When I visited a friend in New York she told me about playing with her visiting grandson. One day, they tried bending over to see if they could touch their toes. Her grandson pointed out that while my friend bent over far (which is very good because she is in her sixties) he noticed that her upper back fell over in a chunk. My friend is very limber in her hips and lower back, but when I watched her bend over I could see what her grandson meant. She curled her spine smoothly, with control and a sense of awareness until she was half-way over, then her upper back fell over in a dense chunk.

My friend and her grandson's very loose version of Standing Forward Bend illustrates the value of yoga. Yoga postures highlight areas that are out of balance, often drawing your attention to them as if they were lit up in neon lights. My friend has an overly extended lower back and an overly contracted her upper back.

To look at her, you would not know that, yet when she assumed a yoga-type posture, it became so obvious that her ten-year-old grandson noticed it immediately. Yoga is a tool for systematically bringing the body back into balance and alignment. It makes dead zones very noticeable.

You have to know there is a problem and where it is before you know how to fix it.

Although I love both of my parents, I hope I won't age like them. That is one reason I practice so diligently. My family chunks up and loses height at a faster rate than most people do.

Older people stand and walk differently than younger people. But I think it is wise to examine what is and what is not an inevitable part of the aging process. Zhu says opening up the joints in qi gong is the secret to the unobstructed flow of qi and of good health.

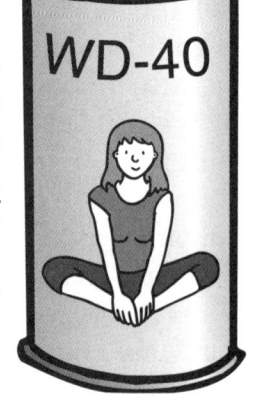

Yoga and qi gong are like much-needed WD-40 for your joints.

Zhu has his students do hip circles to help open up the joints in the body. He can do thousands of hip circles at a time "no problem." He says that he uses his mind to control this, not his muscles. Whirling dervishes come to my mind when he says this; there has to be something other than pure muscle involved to spin with their speed and intensity.

Evaluate your joint mobility.

Hip Circles Exercise

1. Stand with your feet hip distance apart and parallel to each other.

2. Move your hips in clockwise circles as shown in the diagram. The view is looking down from the top of your body.

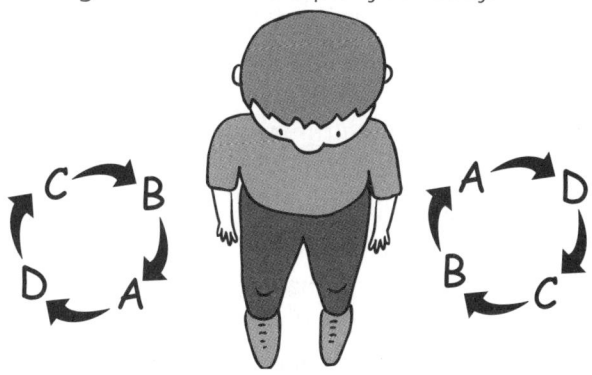

3. When your left hip is at point A in its circle, your right hip should also be at point A in its circle. Your feet remain relaxed and long along their length on the floor, your head up and looking straight ahead.

4. Complete a minimum of 25 circles.

5. Repeat with counterclockwise circles.

This exercise will affect all of the joints of your body, from your ankles all the way up to your neck and shoulders.

Were you able to easily make smooth, round circles? Students in class sometimes feel that instead of circles they are making triangles or even straight lines because their range of motion is so limited.

Journal Entry

As I stepped outside this morning, I listened to the chatter of the birds back from their winter trip south. Their chatter filled the air as I started working in the yard. When I came back into the house, I realized that after just a few moments outside I had stopped noticing the bird sounds. Their voices, which still filled the air, no longer entered my conscious awareness. How quickly my attention had wandered away from my surroundings. Meditation has

*made me aware of how quickly I lose focus and of how I can be so
unaware of what is internally happening in my body.*

*Five minutes into my first seated meditation I started squirm-
ing, vaguely aware of some discomfort along my midriff. As I
continued to sit I was able to pinpoint a constriction there. The
bottom of my rib cage felt as if it was surrounded by a tight, thick
rubber band. That tight, thick rubber band was my diaphragm.*

*The instant I finished meditating my discomfort vanished; it
receded from my conscious awareness as easily as the voices of the
birds outside had. Somehow I disconnect myself from the pain of
my rubber-band tight diaphragm.*

*Meditative perspective awakened me to the habitual tightness
in my diaphragm. It added a new dimension of understanding.
The experience was similar to the one of looking at one of those
pictures out of which a three-dimensional picture emerges when
you change the focus of your gaze.*

*Debra Ann says that meditation is not hard, it is not about
accomplishing anything or becoming something you are not. The
meditative state is the natural way to be. You have to let go of the
obstacles that keep you from it. The obstacles are your attachments. Meditation helps you observe your thoughts and the
attachments you form from them. Your attachments to your
thoughts cause anxiety, anxiety leads to problems like a rubber-
band diaphragm.*

*I still think meditation is hard. Learning to be natural is hard
work.*

Yoga practice teaches you to how to observe and relax your anxious thoughts. You gain a more neutral perspective. A meditative
outlook does not change your inherent characteristics, it trains you
to let go of the obstacles that cloud and obscure them. An ideal body
image is just one such obstacle.

It is often easier to ignore our discomfort than it is to face the
fear that put it there. This is why we block out the discomfort. This
is why we often don't follow through on our resolutions. We even
forget what it is we resolved to do.

Have you ever resolved to change something in your life once and
for all and then three weeks later you belatedly remember your resolve?

Sitting Meditation

Beginning meditation:

1. Sit in a comfortable chair with your feet flat on the floor and your hands resting lightly on your thighs.

2. Soften your gaze by imagining that your eyes are located at the back of your head.

3. Breathe normally for five minutes.

4. Focus your attention at the tip of your nostrils where your breath enters and leaves your body.

5. Keep your attention focused on your nostrils and pay attention to your next inhalation from its beginning to its end.

6. Keep the thread of the memory of your inhalation as it flows into your exhalation.

7. Pay attention to your next exhalation from its beginning to its end.

8. Keep the thread of the memory of your exhalation as it flows into your next inhalation.

9. Repeat this for ten minutes.

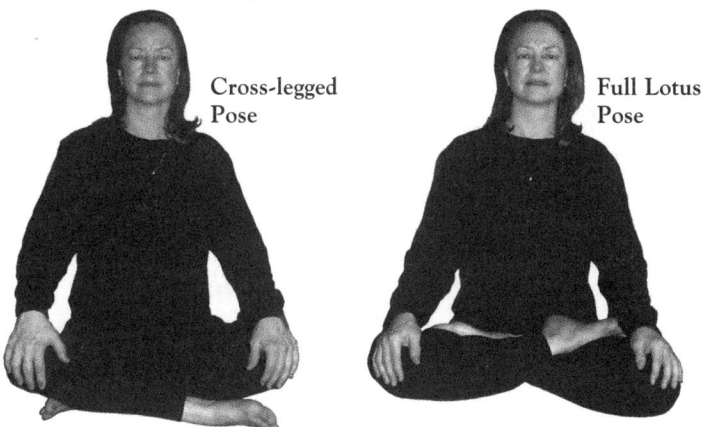

Cross-legged Pose

Full Lotus Pose

As your flexibility increases, you can try this in Cross-legged Pose or Full Lotus Pose.

What was the quality of your thoughts during this exercise? Did they interfere with your concentration on your breath?

Did you notice anything else?

Journal Entry

I sometimes fantasize what it would be like to feel my twenty-five-year-old body again, replaced with my fifty-year-old brain, of course. I wouldn't mind borrowing my sixty-five-year-old brain for a while, assuming I will continue to shore up more wisdom as I age. Maybe I will let my hair go naturally gray; maybe I'll do it just so that I know I can. I don't have to keep it gray if I don't like it. There's always Charlie to turn to. Maybe I will let my hair go gray on my sixty-fifth birthday.

Came across notes from a visualization I did during my summer of tennis. I was told that you look over your left shoulder to access your past and you look over your right shoulder to access your future. Looking back over my left shoulder, I had visualized my younger self as a princess with a long flowing gown against a gold-toned background. Looking back over my right shoulder I had visualized my older self as an old crone dressed in a black cape with a witchlike nose against a dark background.

I know I have changed a lot. Tried the same visualization today. Did some deep, even breathing first so I could stay as focused as possible in the present moment. Closed my eyes and concentrated on images from the past, until I felt I had the essence of my younger self. Then concentrated on visualizing myself aging, my face becoming more lined, my hair turning from gray to white. I felt anxious at first as I imagined myself getting older. I located the essence of my older self. I brought the two essences together within my heart so that I could nurture them both equally.

Somewhat paradoxically, while yoga and qi gong help you look and feel younger, they also help you accept the aging process. You develop a trust that you are the best that you can be. You look out from the center of your experience and from that center you don't worry so much about the changes that occur with aging. The center is located in the present moment of existence.

The daily practice of focusing on what is happening in the present during your practice helps you to do so more frequently during the rest of the day. Your natural body shape exists in the present and changes. It changes from one moment to the next. The closest, most fully rewarding relationship you can have with your body is to be aware of it fully each moment of your existence. When you focus on this present moment, the past and future merge into it.

Old Self/Young Self Exercise

1. Close your eyes. Look back over your left shoulder.
2. Picture yourself at a younger age.
3. Close your eyes and look back over your right shoulder.
4. Picture yourself much older than you are now. What does this older person have to offer you?
5. Bring the two images together in your heart.

Journal Entry

> Released the density in my upper chest and shoulders, in standing meditation. The density dissolves into stability in my legs. I feel much stronger in the pose. Releasing the density in my upper chest and shoulders changes my center of gravity, I think. My neck and head straighten up of their own accord, and I feel comfortable in the new alignment. This new alignment is not yet permanent, but it will be one day.
>
> I am slowly learning to relax my chest and shoulders so that they are supported naturally by my hips and legs. When I look in the mirror, the curve of my neck is beginning to more closely resemble the natural curve of the spine.
>
> The release of density in my chest changes the energy flow in my body. Zhu talks a lot about energy flow when he teaches qi gong.

To picture what density in the chest looks like, take a look at the Forward Bends in diagrams A and B. Diagram A depicts the form of a woman from one of my yoga books. In practice I have rarely seen anyone in my yoga classes, even the teachers, this flexible. The second diagram shows an example of density in the chest; notice the

Diagram A   Diagram B

145

arrow. Can you see the difference?

Even though both torsos lie against the thighs, one has better energy flow than the other does.

Density occurs when energy flow is blocked. And blocked energy flow means decreased energy for the creative aspects of your life. Blocked energy creates an unaligned body. Remember that 85 percent of our energy is expended holding ourselves upright against gravity. We think of gravity as a force that weighs us down, makes our bodies sag, makes it more difficult to walk. A body with no energy blocks, one that is aligned with the gravitational field, is light. A body with no energy blocks ages more slowly and gracefully.

The basic posture of qi gong is standing mediation. Thousands of Chinese do this meditation in the parks in China daily. This meditation will gradually work through the energy blocks in your body, one block at a time.

Standing Meditation Exercise

Standing meditation looks deceptively simple. One friend who thought he was in good physical shape couldn't bend at the hips enough to hold the posture for three minutes. Zhu can do standing meditation for two hours "no problem." He says that he experiences a buoyant "up" energy that flows through and supports him. He says that this "up" energy flows when one has worked through the energy blocks (that result in tight muscles, twisted spine, stiff joints, and so forth) and is completely relaxed and aligned in the pose.

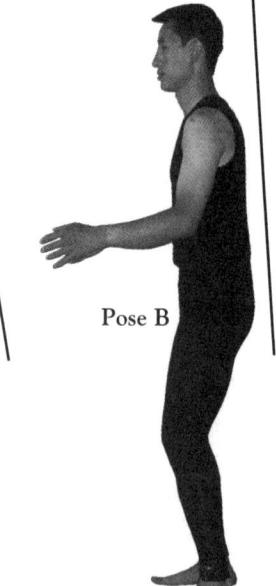

Pose A

Pose B

1. Stand with your feet hip-distance apart and parallel to each other.

2. "Sit down" into an imaginary chair.

3. Your spine should be straight.

146

4. Your knees should be aligned over the middle of your toes.

5. If you are very flexible you will end up in pose A, otherwise you sink down as far as you can, keeping your spine straight, ending up closer to pose B.

6. Relax your whole body, starting from your feet all the way to the top of your head over and over again.

7. Imagine yourself being suspended from a point above the crown of your head.

8. Stay in the pose for thirty minutes.

I think of this pose as a sitting version of yoga's Mountain Pose. You can also try standing in Mountain Pose for five or ten minutes before you bend your knees and sit.

Journal Entry

Dug out my bathing suit so I could go to the lake. I think I will need a new suit soon. Finding the right bathing suit for the few occasions I need to wear one can take years. I dressed quickly and left the house. When I removed my shorts and glanced down at my stomach I discovered with awe that it looked different in my suit. It was smaller and softer than I remembered it to be the last time. It looked a little like a deflated balloon but not flabby.

I hadn't noticed this change. I have spent my whole life struggling to fix my stomach and then miss a significant transformation. I guess one reason for the oversight is that I have turned off the glaring spotlight.

The most satisfying transformation for me has been the difference in the shape of my stomach. The difference in its shape reflects the difference in my relationship with my body and my life.

Your natural body shape evolves over time. Through daily discipline, your relationship with your body deepens into mutual understanding, love, and trust. You cannot develop this understanding and trust with dislike, when you are at odds with it. Your body can learn to respond to whatever you want it to do. You will be more accepting of its weaknesses and strengths, working with both to the best of your ability.

CHAPTER 13

The Little Buddha Test

Journal Entry

    I watched preview ads for the movie Moulin Rouge. *One shot highlighted Nicole Kidman's gorgeous legs. I started my grocery store dialogue—I wish my legs looked like that, I need to jog more, do my calf exercises more regularly—until I became aware of my thoughts. This is the part where meditation practice comes in. Meditation teaches you how to observe your thoughts away from your emotional attachment to them. What on earth would I do with thirty-something legs on my fifty-four-year-old body? And really, I have always liked my legs.*

    As I let go of the fears that create an ideal image, I become free of it. The emotions created by my attachment to the image pull and tug and create turmoil within me; they are the vortex of my kaleidoscope dream. The more I acknowledge and work through my fears, the closer I am to peace.

In a scene from the movie *Little Buddha*, Siddhartha sits in meditation. As Siddhartha sits, Maya, the God of Illusion of this world, challenges him. Maya conjures up beautiful women, tidal waves, and even Siddhartha's own self-image in order to distract him. But Siddhartha is in the process of becoming enlightened. He stays fo-

148

cused in his meditation and is not moved by any of these images because he knows they are illusions.

The first time I saw the movie I thought Siddhartha had to have a will of iron to resist the powerful illusions. However, he is not resisting. He has let go of his attachments and Maya's illusions have no power over him. He sits in meditation with ease.

Media images can teach you about yourself. The more you learn to observe your thoughts in a meditative way, the more you will be able to see the images for the illusions they are. Meditation teaches you not to try to make your thoughts disappear; the more you try to do that, the stronger their influence becomes. The story is of the student who tells his teacher that he cannot get rid of his thoughts. The teacher tells him it is okay to think of any thought except monkeys. Of course, the student goes back to meditate and all he can think of is monkeys.

When you are in harmony with your natural body shape you don't have to ignore media images, or love or hate them. You begin to see them for what they are. Whatever form Maya, the God of Illusion, takes—a gorgeous model in a magazine, a current fashion trend that leaves your body type out, or even a fashion trend that exemplifies your body type—you recognize your responses to them. They become like the thoughts you observe in sitting meditation.

The more secure you are in the wisdom and strength of your own natural body, the more the vortex of strong emotions created by illusions disappears and you have nothing left to struggle with. Such an enlightened response does not happen overnight; you continually observe yourself and your reactions, learning from what they have to teach.

Societal and media images have their place in our culture. When you become secure within your own body your responses are healthier. You use whatever helpful hints are available from the pictures and people around you. Maybe a model in a magazine is wearing a color or jewelry that would look good on you. To react in this way is healthy, wanting to look your best. You build your unique look based upon your body's natural shape.

What you take from media images is not the desire to have a body different from what you have, but helpful input to make you look your best. Your sense of your natural shape comes from within you, not from magazines or TV, however you take from them what you can use. Talented and artistic people create the pictures in magazines and on television. It would be a shame not to take advantage of their expertise.

A strong self-image goes beyond how you respond to current body fashion trends. A strong self-image changes your whole life.

Little Buddha Exercise

The next time you peruse a magazine or any time you come across images of what you consider to be the body beautiful, focus on your breathing.

1. Pay attention to your thoughts and the feelings that go along with them.

2. Release any anxiety with the exhalation of your breath.

3. Look to see if the image has any helpful hints for you.

4. If your reaction is happiness that your body looks really great, that is fine, but also be comfortable with how it might change and be different tomorrow.

Journal Entry

Missed practice for two days and had very short practices for another eight days during the Christmas holiday. I was dismayed at how anxious I started to feel about my appearance again. I had lost some of my inner poise, something I had begun to take for granted. It returned once I resumed my regular practice.

Practice helps me to access a place within that is quiet and calm. This place is my spot in the universe. I don't have to be anyone other than myself. I don't have to strive for anything in the world because everything without is already within. It keeps me on an even keel. I don't have to manipulate the outer events of my life because I can handle whatever happens from the calm within. I don't have to worry about how I look or what I am doing because I am doing the best I can.

The strongest, most flexible student in my yoga class today has a round stomach. So do most of the other female students, *which is most of the class. My stomach is naturally round. Round is beautiful. Round is plentiful. I remember when I controlled my eating enough to have a flat stomach. I ate very little and my friends and family cautioned that I was too thin. I was too thin.*

When my stomach was flat, my thighs started to really bother me. The only time they ever did. In the spotlight of my disapproval, they looked too flabby. Once I returned to a more normal weight and my stomach rounded out I turned my spotlight back on it. To me this reinforces the notion that the dislike I have had for my body came from my own self-doubt and a lack of self-acceptance. If one part of my body got "fixed," I transferred my feelings to a different part.

I have a new sense of myself. I have worked through a lot of my feelings and have greater inner poise. Inner poise is what the Little Buddha test is all about.

Do I mourn my fallen ideal body image?

I don't.

Diet, exercise and cosmetic surgery will not make my body perfect.

I will never have Julie Christie's nose (she will undoubtedly be relieved).

My stomach will never look like the stomach of a lingerie model or department store mannequin.

It doesn't matter so much anymore.

What a relief.

Enlightenment sounds great. But it is a struggle to get to the state of nonstruggle. To learn equanimity, to be able to accept and handle life's different events and outcomes with detachment and courage is the primary goal that makes sense to me. Attachment causes pain, my teachers remind me over and over again, as their teachers remind them. I imagine the Little Buddha test is the bottom-line test for a positive self-image. The ability to look at all of the images Maya, in the form of our society, conjures before you, and to be calm in your wisdom is an enlightened way to be.

Instead of coping with your aging body, accept and make your aging body the best that it can be. Anti-aging is a struggle against the inevitable. Aging well and gracefully is not.

CHAPTER 14

Ageless Grace

Journal Entry

I am glad I have traded an ideal image for being more naturally who I am. I continue to reap priceless rewards and compliments for the way I look. For example, I was having a treatment at David, my chiropractor's office one day. David is a network chiropractor, and uses a technique that twitches and tweaks you and can look very odd to a casual observer, but it is intended to help the body figure out its own mind/body connection. Sometimes he needs help to hold your body in certain positions during a session.

His new assistant was asked to help position my body for part of a treatment. Afterward, in the outer office, she asked me what I did to have the body I have. She has been looking into yoga and I encouraged her to find a good teacher and take classes.

My friend Delores complimented me in an unusual way, from an almost fall. I was visiting her in San Diego. I stepped on an uneven section of sidewalk, one with a small hole, and almost fell (Bob says that if there is a hole in the sidewalk to fall into, I will find it). As I saved myself from the fall, Delores was impressed— you did that so gracefully, she exclaimed. I think I know what she meant. As I lost my balance I immediately took pressure off of my bent ankle, saving it from being sprained or even broken. I simultaneously had mind awareness in other parts of my body, adjusting them to minimize any injury to me. This is mind/body connection *at work. The sensation I had was of my body adjusting itself as I orchestrated the show.*

Journal Entry

Every morning I affirm that I am my natural body shape height and that I have regained the natural curve and health of my spine. A pharmacy student Bob met at a party told him that Americans in their fifties and older are most often taking some form of mood altering medication or herb. Bob and I take no prescription or over the counter drugs.

Several of my friends struggle with depression and are on medication for that. One friend described his experience with an antidepressant. He said that on the drug his thoughts are still there but the heaviness is gone from them. Sounds like meditation to me. Another friend stopped taking this medication because she said it made her feel like a zombie. You don't get that side effect from meditation.

My mood shifters are my practice. One day after doing a standing meditation in the afternoon, I felt a huge release of heat and tension from my shoulders and upper chest. I felt limp, but happy, like I had just been given a tremendous workout from a massage. One morning a yoga class of backbends left me feeling euphoric for the rest of the day. The teacher pointed out this benefit during the class.

Yoga postures balance hormonal and glandular secretions. They bring nourishment to the organs and glands by bathing them in blood.

In his book *The Concise Light on Yoga*, Mr. Iyengar says that in shoulder stand "There are several endocrine organs or ductless glands in the human system which bathe in blood, absorb the nutrients from the blood and secrete hormones for the proper functioning of a balanced and well-developed body and brain." He goes on to say, "Amazingly enough many of the *asanas* [postures] have a direct effect on the glands and help them to function properly. *Sarvangasana* [shoulder stand] does this for the thyroid and parathyroid glands which are situated in the neck region, since due to the firm chin lock their blood supply is increased."

Words really cannot describe the depth of benefits you get from daily practice of these arts. You have to try it for yourself.

After having set myself adrift in the wilderness, I have discovered that I am not rudderless without an ideal image. I have my intent that guides me, my faith in the principles of the teachings of my practice. I test them out and as they work I gain more faith in their truth, in their ability to help me lead the life I want. So while I initially felt as if I had taken a plunge into dangerous rapids, my practice is like a strong oar that guides me safely through. It shows me the underlying, calm current beneath the rapids. What I do comes from the inner wisdom I develop, not from without, although without are the events that help me to gain that wisdom, to see where I am strong and where I am weak, to mirror back my soul to me.

Siddhartha's source of calm is his understanding of the nature of reality. Therefore, he can't be fooled by Maya. The nature of reality is expansive, I think. Debra Ann talks about experiencing the vastness and boundlessness of existence through yoga. Zhu talks about moving qi by placing his mind outside of his body and of his experience of a flow of energy that is opposite from gravity. This antigravity energy is the "up" energy that supports him for hours in standing meditation pose.

Conclusion

As I write this conclusion it is the winter of 2002. I can hardly believe I have spent nine years writing my book. I wondered if a lot of what I had written in the beginning would seem outdated. Then I came across a book in the library called *Ophelia Speaks* by Sara Shandler. *Ophelia Speaks* is a book about teenage girls and their struggles with their search for self. In the beginning several of them talk about their body images.

An eighteen-year-old stands before a mirror and looks at her reflection with disgust. She hates her body and herself. Along the frame of her mirror are photographs of the models she wants to look like. One fifteen-year-old sits with her friend and observes as her friend flips through a catalog, cooing at a "Barbie doll model" (her words) in a catalog. The book was published in 1999. I don't think much has changed at all.

The author of this book says that when she sent out invitations to teenage girls to write their contributions, she never suggested "The Media" as a topic. Yet nearly twenty girls sent in essays blaming the media for their poor body image. I understand their frustration. They probably feel boxed in and caged, with no way out.

Neill and I went to the zoo to see the new "open area" primate exhibit. The area was gorgeous but we didn't see any animals in it. After looking at the exhibit we sat down and ate ice cream. I thought about the gorillas in their new cage, a larger more "open-spaced" area, but still a cage.

I thought about us, living on earth, in a larger, more expansive cage than the one that the gorillas inhabit. Life does feel like a cage at times, but whatever is beyond this realm of my existence is just as unavailable to me as the rest of the earth is unavailable to the gorillas. If there are other dimensions and realms beyond this one, I am too limited to experience them right now.

The ideal body image has been a cage I have created and imprisoned myself in for most of my life. No wonder I feel such empathy for the gorillas. My friend Marilyn tells me that the Sufis believe human beings are in a cage but that its door is not locked; most of us just don't realize we could open the door and walk out at any time. I guess that being in a cage brought on by our perceptions is a widespread philosophical concept. I didn't know that. I mostly read murder mysteries. Maybe I should expand my reading list.

But the earth experience is one of lessons to be learned, I believe. My ideal image has taught me a lot about myself. I have used it as a tool for self-exploration and growth. What I have learned the most from have been the hardest challenges in life.

If I could, I would tell these young teenagers that your body is your spiritual teacher. From it you can learn your greatest strengths and your greatest weaknesses, as well as everything in between. You can learn how to cultivate and utilize your strengths and strengthen your weaknesses. Your strengths can help teach your weaknesses.

Taking yoga is one route to this end. Yoga teaches self-observation. Be aware of what you are feeling when you look at gorgeous models in magazines Acknowledge your feelings, and take responsibility for them. Whether you are feeling angry, jealous, discouraged, or even prideful, these emotions are your tools for self-examination. Even if you are happy that your body looks a lot like a model in a magazine, let that feeling go, too. Remember that fashion trends can change, and what is in one day may be out the next. If your happiness with yourself is based upon that resemblance, what happens if the pictures change next year? What if you change next year?

Use the media images to your advantage. When you do, you can look at these pictures dispassionately, maybe a model is wearing a color that looks good on you, or maybe a clothes combination you could use. You do not become a zombie, but you react in a way that is centered and appropriate. If a picture has nothing to offer you, move on. I now notice how exceedingly thin are the arms and shoulders of the lingerie models with flat stomachs. A lot of them don't look very well nourished. I hope you are well nourished.

While I have used media images as a prime example, I think that we have to be aware of how the reactions of the people in our lives, our friends, our spouses, our children, our partners, our lovers, all can play the same kind of role.

A client of mine once came in full of both happiness and anxiety. She was so happy that everything in her life was going so well. She was anxious and scared because she was afraid that things would change. I tried to reassure her. I didn't have enough wisdom then to tell her that what she feared would inevitably happen. Her life would change. Buddhists say that the defining nature of our reality is its impermanence.

To handle that impermanence well:

- Face your fears.
- Face your angers.
- Take responsibility for everything you experience.
- Practice doing all of the above every day.

I have written that I am not so sure we should spend our time and energy focusing on changing media images. The route to a happy, healthy body image is through self-exploration and transformation. That is an unbeatable formula for success. The only person you have to worry about changing, the only person you really can change, is you.

The value of yoga and qi gong in the transformation of self is that they are the tools that can guide you to create the healthy relationship with your body that you want. With daily practice they can give you, as they have given me, a view of your body that is much more rewarding than an ideal body that can never be real.

A cage surrounds our hearts. We seem born with the need to protect it from harm. The tricky aspect of this is that we need to protect ourselves when necessary and yet allow ourselves to be open to the love and support of others.

The journey to a natural body shape is a journey of the heart. When we learn self-acceptance we learn to accept others as well. The process of softening the heart and the rib cage changes the way you view yourself and others. It demands focus and attention, like any other yogic or qi gong process. It brings you into the present, working with the body you have, its pains and limitations as well as its strengths and weaknesses. You establish a working relationship with what is real. You feel kinder toward yourself. The ideal body image does not wrinkle, does not feel pain, and is stiff and wooden in its perfection. It must be an illusion.

The natural body shape evolves from the daily habit of practice. You struggle to let go of the fears and judgments that prevent you from loving and accepting yourself rather than letting those fears and judgments construct an image you cannot live up to. This is the fundamental difference between the natural body shape and the ideal body image.

I have finally obtained a copy of the book that talks about creating an imaginary council of advisors: *Think and Grow Rich* by Napoleon Hill. His imaginary council comes at the very end of the book and he says it is the last step, given you have mastered all of the steps that precede it. Now I know why my caged girl spoke up, she was an uncompleted step. His book is a classic and I recommend it as a guide for growing rich in self-acceptance and healthy body attitude.

I hope that it is time for a revolution in body image. A revolution that evolves from inside and radiates outward, with appropriate actions coming from a sense of clear identity and strong self-image.

The following two final exercises are exercises for opening the heart and for cultivating loving kindness.

Heart Exercise

To release tension and open up the heart area. Yoga blankets are made of wool or wool and synthetic blends and they are about 6-feet square. Use a blanket that is soft and feels comfortable.

1. *Roll up the blanket so that it is about 4 inches thick, and place it on the floor.*

2. *Position yourself so that the blanket will lie underneath your shoulder blades when you lie in Corpse Pose.*

3. Roll down from a seated position and bring your arms out at a 45-degree angle from your torso. Turn your palms up toward the ceiling.

4. You can adjust the thickness of the blanket if it feels too high or too low once you put it underneath you (see picture).

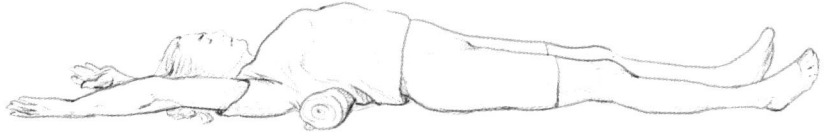

5. Relax completely into the blanket. Focus on your breath, inhale and exhale slowly and steadily.

6. Do this for five minutes. Then gently sit up.

Loving Kindness Meditation

1. Sit comfortably in a chair with your hands on your thighs.

2. Breathe normally for a few moments.

3. Close your eyes.

4. Focus your attention on your breath and take slow, deep inhalations and exhalations.

5. Find your spot in the universe.

6. Then wish yourself the following:

> May I be happy,
> May I be free from anger, worry and fear.
> May I come into the light.
> May I be complete.
> May I be happy.

7. Create the feeling of love and happiness you wish for yourself within.

8. Let this feeling spread out from your heart:

> May all sentient beings be happy.

Epilogue

Journal Entry

National Public Radio (NPR) said today that scientists study-ing supernovas had discovered a mysterious energy that works against gravity. I immediately thought of Zhu's experience of "up" energy in standing meditation.

It is hard for me to explain "up" energy because I haven't devel-oped my practice to the point where I can access and use it (if I ever will).

Use of the "up" energy was demonstrated in a Bill Moyers tape from his series "Healing and the Mind." A T'ai Chi master lines up his students in a chain, each one touching the student in front and in back. The master proceeds to apparently lightly touch the first student and like dominos, all of the students fall down. The master on this tape is one of Zhu's teachers (you can see a picture of Zhu on the tape). With no frame of reference to understand how this could happen, one might think there has to be some trick involved or that the students are making themselves fall down.

But I know otherwise: Zhu can move qi energy. Before we met Zhu, Bob and I studied T'ai Chi with Bing. Bing enjoyed knocking his students down with the touch of his hand, just like the T'ai Chi master on Bill Moyers tape did. One time Bob and I were having lunch in the restaurant owned by Bing's family. I asked Bing to show me what the "force" felt like. He did. One moment I was standing, the next moment I was on the floor. He didn't hurt me. I crumpled

160

to the ground feeling like he had disconnected some circuit within me. So to me, the "up" energy is a fact of life.

Zhu's mysterious "up" energy and the universal flow of qi are unfamiliar concepts to most Westerners. I tried to explain this to a friend I was visiting in New York. She shook her head. Even though she knew me to be intelligent and rational, she could not fit what I was telling her into her framework of experience. This doesn't mean it's not real, one needs to expand one's frame of reference in order to understand how these energies work.

Author B. K. Frantzis spent many years studying a variety of martial arts in China. In his book, *Opening the Energy Gates of Your Body*, he describes his first meeting with a qi gong master. Mr. Frantzis, an experienced martial artist himself at the time, using all of his power and skill, was unable to budge the little finger of the master. Zhu says that is because the master aligned himself with the universal flow of qi, to move him would be like trying to move the whole universe.

Most of us have no intention of becoming martial artists. However, imagine being able to align with and utilize the universal flow of energy. This qi energy that the qi gong master uses to demonstrate his skills can also be used to cultivate good health, healing, and longevity. Most people practice qi gong for these reasons.

I don't know if Bob and I will ever develop the X-ray vision into the energy patterns of the body of people like Debra Ann and Zhu. Our insight has improved over the years as we continue our own practices. We were having dinner with a friend at a restaurant and Bob pointed out the posture of a young waitress. As he did so I could feel my body contract at the tailbone, tipping my pelvis back, as hers was. I observed the energy pattern of her body by a response within my own. The flow of energy that seemed so mysterious ten years ago has become something familiar to us.

Journal Entry

Scientists are discovering more and more information about the genes that make up our hereditary characteristics.

When my mother was ill and I moved my parents closer to us, I had the unenviable job of packing up their house. My mother saved everything. Downstairs in the basement I came across boxes and boxes of creative projects in various stages of completion—knitting, sewing, painting—that belonged to my mother, my sister, and me. If there is a gene that finishes projects that you start, my family must have that one turned off. My father didn't have any hobbies. Maybe he recognized futility when he saw it.

Bob gave me a book called *The Tao of Chaos* by Katya Walker. In it she describes her experience in the remarkably appropriate responses to what was going on in her life from the Chinese oracle called the I Ching. You ask it questions and find your answers from its terse hexagrams. (It worked the same type of magic for me.) Dr. Walker has a PhD with postdoctoral experience at the Jung institute in Zurich. In the book she describes the struggle between her rational, analytical training and the results she got from her personal experience.

The result of her conflict was an investigation that uncovered the parallels between its ancient system and Western science. The structure and operation of the I Ching is uncannily similar to that of our genetic DNA. What if this is a communication link to our genes? I hope so. Then I can turn on my project gene and finish everything I start.

Yogis talk about experiencing a reality beyond time in their meditation practices. If there is such a realm, then my abyss is truly an illusion.

Beyond just a physically and mentally healthy body as we know it, who knows what other vast possibilities exist for the human mind and body?

Index of Poses

*Bold type indicates the page on which instructions for the pose can be found.

About the Models

Ashlee Dunn teaches yoga at Gentle Strength Yoga Studio in Greenwood Village, and at Denver Ashtanga Yoga Center.

Debra Ann Robinson has private sessions in her Denver home. She gives instruction in yoga, the yoga sutras, and meditation.

Jeanne Ann Walter is an owner of and teaches yoga at Colorado School of Yoga in Denver.

Lura Williams is a student who has practiced yoga regularly since 1995.

Steve Koehler teaches yoga at Gentle Strength Yoga Studio in Greenwood Village.

Suzanna Del Vecchio teaches yoga at Colorado School of Yoga and at The Moving Arts Cooperative Studio in Denver.

Zhu Xilin teaches qi gong classes at The Moving Arts Cooperative Studio in Denver and at Kakes Studio in Boulder.

Bibliography

Albom, Mitch, *Tuesdays with Morrie: An Old Man, a Young Man, and Life's Greatest Lesson*, Doubleday, 1997.

Anderson, Bob, *Stretching: For Everyday Fitness and for Running, Tennis, Racquetball, Cycling, Swimming, Golf, and Other Sports*, Shelter Publications, Inc., 1980.

Choudhury, Bikram, *Bikram's Beginning Yoga Class*, Putnam, 1978.

Delany, Sarah and A. Elizabeth, with Amy Hill Hearth, *Having Our Say: The Delany Sisters' First 100 years*, Kodansha America, Inc., 1993.

Fielding, Helen, *Bridget Jones's Diary*, Viking Penguin, 1998.

Frantzis, B. K., *Opening the Energy Gates of Your Body*, North Atlantic Books, 1993.

Hanna, Thomas, *Somatics: Reawakening the Mind's Control of Movement, Flexibility, and Health*, Addison-Wesley Publishing Company, 1992.

Hill, Napoleon, *Think and Grow Rich*, Fawcett Books, 1990.

Iyengar, B .K. S., *The Concise Light on Yoga*, Schocken Books, 1982.

Jeffers, Susan, *Feel the Fear and Do It Anyway*, Fawcett Books, 1992.

Lerner, Harriett, *The Dance of Anger*, HarperCollins, 1997.

Moody, Harry R., *The Five Stages of the Soul*, Doubleday, 1998.

Nelson, Portia, *There's a Hole in My Sidewalk: The Romance of Self-Discovery*, Beyond Words Publishing, Inc., 1993.

Rolf, Ida Pauline, *Ida Rolf Talks About Rolfing and Physical Reality*, HarperCollins, 1976.

Shandler, Sara, *Ophelia Speaks: Adolescent Girls Write About Their Search for Self*, HarperPerennial, 1999.

Give the Gift of

Natural Body, Natural Shape

to Your Friends and Colleagues

CHECK YOUR LEADING BOOKSTORE OR ORDER HERE

❑ **YES**, I want _____ copies of *Natural Body, Natural Shape* at $14.95 each, plus $4.95 shipping per book (Colorado residents please add $1.08 sales tax per book). Canadian orders must be accompanied by a postal money order in U.S. funds. Allow 15 days for delivery.

❑ **YES**, I am interested in having Barbara B. Moroney speak or give a seminar to my company, association, school, or organization. Please send information.

My check or money order for $_____ is enclosed.

Please charge my: ❑ Visa ❑ MasterCard
  ❑ Discover ❑ American Express

Name _____

Organization _____

Address _____

City/State/Zip _____

Phone_____ E-mail _____

Card # _____

Exp. Date_____ Signature _____

Please make your check payable and return to:
Swing-Hi Press
16213 E. Mercer Circle • Aurora, CO 80013

Call your credit card order to: 866-828-8725
Fax: 303-766-2989

www.naturalbodyshape.com